ICD-10 ...
Psychiatry

A learning guide

Dr Jaspreet Phull
MBChB MRCPsych DipMedSci
Consultant Forensic Psychiatrist
Nottingham

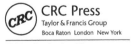

CRC Press
Taylor & Francis Group
Boca Raton London New York

CRC Press is an imprint of the
Taylor & Francis Group, an **informa** business

CRC Press
Taylor & Francis Group
6000 Broken Sound Parkway NW, Suite 300
Boca Raton, FL 33487-2742

ISBN-13: 978 184619 517 4

Visit the Taylor & Francis Web site at
http://www.taylorandfrancis.com

and the CRC Press Web site at
http://www.crcpress.com

British Library Cataloguing in Publication Data

A catalogue record for this book is available from the British Library.

Typeset by Phoenix Photosetting, Chatham, Kent

Contents

Contents

Preface

During my time revising for my psychiatry postgraduate examinations, I found learning of the ICD-10 for diagnosis particularly testing, especially given the depth and complexity of the criteria.

I found aide-mémoires in the form of mnemonics particularly helpful to support my learning of the subject, allowing for much more efficient recall.

Core to psychiatry is the practice of assessment, diagnosis and management. This process is dependent upon a robust knowledge of the diagnostic criteria influencing the clinical management of individuals with a mental disorder.

This guide is not intended to be entirely comprehensive and should be used in conjunction with other ICD-10 resource books. I would recommend this book to those who have an interest in learning about diagnostic coding in psychiatry, including: medical students, psychiatry trainees, mental health professionals and anyone who has an interest in the subject matter.

I would like to thank the World Health Organization for allowing me to reproduce and use its diagnostic criteria.

Jaspreet Phull
January 2012

About the author

Jaspreet is a consultant forensic psychiatrist, practising in Nottingham. Jaspreet studied medicine and qualified from Bristol University in 2003 and gained his MRCPsych qualification in 2007.

His interest in forensic psychiatry stems from his childhood and he has passionately followed his dreams. He has published a number of articles within his specialty but this is his first book. Jaspreet lives with his wife, baby son and two dogs in Lincolnshire, and looks forward to the arrival of his second child next year.

Dedicated to my family:
my wife and bump, son, mama, papa, brother and his family.

The structure of the ICD-10 classification for mental and behavioural disorders

Summary of the diagnostic groups within the ICD-10

Diagnostic categories

F00–F09	Organic, including symptomatic, mental disorders
F10–F19	Mental and behavioural disorders due to psychoactive substance use
F20–F29	Schizophrenia, schizotypal and delusional disorders
F30–F39	Mood (affective) disorders
F40–F48	Neurotic, stress-related and somatoform disorders
F50–F59	Behavioural syndromes associated with physiological disturbances and physical factors
F60–F69	Disorders of adult personality and behaviour
F70–F79	Mental retardation (Learning disability)
F80–F89	Disorders of psychological development
F90–F98	Behavioural and emotional disorders with onset usually occurring in childhood and adolescence
(F99	Mental disorder, unspecified)

O	One = organic
D	Day = drug/alcohol
S	Simon = schizophrenia
M	Made = mood
N	Nick = neurotic
E	Eat = eating and others
P	Pet = personality
L	Lizards = learning disability
D	During = developmental disorder
C	Class = child and adolescence disorders

ODSMNEPLDC = 10 categories

Main diagnoses between categories

1. Organic

F00   Dementia in Alzheimer's disease
F01   Vascular dementia
F02   Dementia in other diseases classified elsewhere
F03   Unspecified dementia (enigmatic)

Dementia in other diseases classified elsewhere
Alzheimer dementia
Vascular dementia
Enigmatic/unspecified dementia
DAVE

Dementias versus non-dementias

F04   Organic amnesic syndrome, not induced by alcohol and other psychoactive substances
F05   Delirium, not induced by alcohol and other psychoactive substances
F06   Other mental disorders due to brain damage and dysfunction and to physical disease
F07   Personality and behavioural disorders due to brain disease, damage and dysfunction
F09   Unspecified organic or symptomatic mental disorder

Mental disorders due to physical disease
Organic amnesic syndrome
Personality and behavioural disorders
Enigmatic/unspecified
Delirium
MOPED

2. Drug/Alcohol

F10.x   Mental and behavioural disorders due to use of alcohol
F11.x   Mental and behavioural disorders due to use of opioids
F12.x   Mental and behavioural disorders due to use of cannabinoids
F13.x   Mental and behavioural disorders due to use of sedatives or hypnotics
F14.x   Mental and behavioural disorders due to use of cocaine
F15.x   Mental and behavioural disorders due to use of other stimulants, including caffeine
F16.x   Mental and behavioural disorders due to use of hallucinogens
F17.x   Mental and behavioural disorders due to use of tobacco

F18.x   Mental and behavioural disorders due to use of volatile solvents

F19.x   Mental and behavioural disorders due to use of multiple drug use and use of other psychoactive substances

Stimulant
Sedative
Solvents (volatile)
Tobacco
Opioids
Multiple psychoactive substance use
Alcohol
Cannabinoids
Cocaine
Hallucinogens
S$_3$TOMAC$_2$H

Subsections

F1x.0   Acute intoxication
F1x.1   Harmful use
F1x.2   Dependence syndrome
F1x.3   Withdrawal state
F1x.4   Withdrawal state with delirium
F1x.5   Psychotic disorder
F1x.6   Amnesic syndrome
F1x.7   Residual disorders and late-onset psychotic disorder
F1x.8   Other mental and behavioural disorders
F1x.9   Unspecified mental and behavioural disorders

This can be divided into: scale of use and effects

Scale of use

Acute Intoxication –> Harmful use –> Dependence

Harmful use
Intoxication
Dependence
HID

Effects

Withdrawal +/- delirium
Amnesia
Residual disorders and late-onset psychotic

Psychotic
'Every other **D**isorder' (F1x.8 + F1x.9)
WARPED

3. Schizophrenia and other disorders

F20   Schizophrenia
F21   Schizotypal disorder
F22   Persistent delusional disorder
F23   Acute and transient psychotic disorders
F24   Induced delusional disorder
F25   Schizoaffective disorders
F28   Other non-organic psychotic disorders
F29   Unspecified non-organic psychosis

Persistent delusional disorder
Acute and transient psychotic disorders
Schizophrenia
Schizo**A**ffective
Generated from another (induced)
Enigmatic (i.e. including other + unspecified non-organic psychotic disorders)
Schizotypal
PASSAGES

4. Mood (affective) disorders

F30   Manic episode
F31   Bipolar affective disorder
F32   Depressive episode
F33   Recurrent depressive disorder
F34   Persistent mood (affective) disorders
F38   Other mood (affective) disorders
F39   Unspecified mood (affective) disorder

Bipolar affective disorder
Unspecified mood disorder
Manic episode
Persistent mood disorders

Recurrent depressive disorder
Other mood disorder
Depressive episode
BUMP ROD

5. Neurotic disorders

F40   Phobic anxiety disorders
F41   Other anxiety disorders
F42   Obsessive-compulsive disorder
F43   Reaction to severe stress, and adjustment disorders
F44   Dissociative (conversion) disorders
F45   Somatoform disorders
F48   Other neurotic disorders

Phobic anxiety disorders
Other anxiety disorders
Obsessive-compulsive disorder
Reaction to severe stress and adjustment disorders

Somatoform disorders
Other neurotic disorders
Dissociative disorders
POOR SOD

6. Behavioural syndromes associated with physiological disturbances and physical factors

F50   Eating disorders
F51   Non-organic sleep disorders
F52   Sexual dysfunction, not caused by organic disorder or disease
F53   Mental and behavioural disorders associated with the puerperium, not elsewhere classified
F54   Psychological and behavioural factors associated with disorders or diseases classified elsewhere
F55   Abuse of non-dependence-producing substances
F59   Unspecified behavioural syndromes associated with physiological disturbances and physical factors

Puerperium-related disorders
Associated elsewhere disorders + unspecified behavioural syndromes
Sleep disorders
Sexual dysfunction
Eating disorders
Drug/medication abuse (that are non-dependence producing)
PASSED

7. Disorders of adult personality and behaviour

F60   Specific personality disorders
F61   Mixed and other personality disorders
F62   Enduring personality changes, not attributable to brain damage and disease

F63	Habit and impulse disorders
F64	Gender identity disorders
F65	Disorders of sexual preference
F66	Psychological and behavioural disorders associated with sexual development and orientation
F68	Other disorders of adult personality and behaviour
F69	Unspecified disorder of adult personality and behaviour

Personality disorders (specific + mixed)
Other disorders of adult personality and behaviour
Psychological and behavioural disorders

Gender identity disorders
Unspecified disorders of adult personality and behaviour
Impulse and habit disorders
Sexual preference disorders
Enduring personality changes
POP GUISE

8. Mental retardation/learning disability

F70	Mild mental retardation (IQ score 50–69)
F71	Moderate mental retardation (IQ score 35–49)
F72	Severe mental retardation (IQ score 20–34)
F73	Profound mental retardation (IQ score <20)
F78	Other mental retardation
F79	Unspecified mental retardation (specifying the extent of associated impairment of behaviour)

Note: Mild –> moderate –> severe –> profound –> other –> unspecified

Other

Mild
Unspecified
Moderate
Profound
Severe
O MUMPS

9. Disorders of psychological development

F80	Specific developmental disorders of speech and language
F81	Specific developmental disorders of scholastic skills
F82	Specific developmental disorder of motor function
F83	Mixed specific developmental disorder
F84	Pervasive developmental disorders
F88	Other disorders of psychological development

F89   Unspecified disorder of psychological development

Pervasive developmental disorder
Other
Scholastic skills
Speech and language
Unspecified disorder
Mixed and Motor
POSSUM$_2$

10. Behavioural and emotional disorders with onset usually occurring in childhood and adolescence

F90   Hyperkinetic disorder
F91   Conduct disorders
F92   Mixed disorders of conduct and emotions
F93   Emotional disorders with onset specific to childhood
F94   Disorders of social functioning with onset specific to childhood and adolescence
F95   Tic disorders
F98   Other behavioural and emotional problems with onset usually occurring in childhood and adolescence

Mixed disorders of conduct and emotions
Emotional disorders with onset specific to childhood
Tic disorders
Hyperkinetic disorder
Other behavioural and emotional problems
Disorders of social functioning
Includes Conduct disorders
METHODIC

11. Unspecified mental disorder
F99   Mental disorder, not otherwise specified

Summary of main diagnostic groups
F00–F09   Organic, including symptomatic, mental disorders = DAVE MOPED
F10–F19   Mental and behavioural disorders due to psychoactive substance use = Categories of substance, Scale of use (HID) + WARPED
F20–F29   Schizophrenia, schizotypal and delusional disorders = PASSAGES
F30–F39   Mood disorders = BUMP ROD
F40–F48   Neurotic, stress-related and somatoform disorders = POOR SOD

F50–F59 Behavioural syndromes associated with physiological disturbances and physical factors = **PASSED**

F60–F69 Disorders of adult personality and behaviour = **POP GUISE**

F70–F79 Mental retardation (learning disability) = **O MUMPS**

F80–F89 Disorders of psychological development = **POSSUM**

F90–F98 Behavioural and emotional disorders with onset usually occurring in childhood and adolescence = **METHODIC**

F99 Unspecified mental disorder

Main ICD-10 diagnostic groups

F00–F09 Organic, including symptomatic, mental disorders
F00 Dementia in Alzheimer's disease
F00.0 Dementia in Alzheimer's disease with early onset
F00.1 Dementia in Alzheimer's disease with late onset
F00.2 Dementia in Alzheimer's disease, atypical or mixed type
F00.9 Dementia in Alzheimer's disease, unspecified

F01 Vascular dementia
F01.0 Vascular dementia of acute onset
F01.1 Multi-infarct dementia
F01.2 Subcortical vascular dementia
F01.3 Mixed cortical and subcortical vascular dementia
F01.8 Other vascular dementia
F01.9 Vascular dementia, unspecified

F02 Dementia in other diseases classified elsewhere
F02.0 Dementia in Pick's disease
F02.1 Dementia in Creutzfeldt–Jakob disease
F02.2 Dementia in Huntington's disease
F02.3 Dementia in Parkinson's disease
F02.4 Dementia in human immunodeficiency virus (HIV) disease
F02.8 Dementia in other specified diseases classified elsewhere

F03 Unspecified dementia
A fifth character may be added to specify dementia in F00–F03, as follows:
.x0 Without additional symptoms
.xl Other symptoms, predominantly delusional
.x2 Other symptoms, predominantly hallucinatory
.x3 Other symptoms, predominantly depressive
.x4 Other mixed symptoms

F04 Organic amnesic syndrome, not induced by alcohol and other psychoactive substances

F05 Delirium, not induced by alcohol and other psychoactive substances
F05.0 Delirium, not superimposed on dementia, so described
F05.1 Delirium, superimposed on dementia
F05.8 Other delirium
F05.9 Delirium, unspecified

F06   Other mental disorders due to brain damage and dysfunction and to physical disease

F06.0   Organic hallucinosis
F06.1   Organic catatonic disorder
F06.2   Organic delusional (schizophrenia-like) disorder
F06.3   Organic mood (affective) disorders:
.30   Organic manic disorder
.31   Organic bipolar affective disorder
.32   Organic depressive disorder
.33   Organic mixed affective disorder
F06.4   Organic anxiety disorder
F06.5   Organic dissociative disorder
F06.6   Organic emotionally labile (asthenic) disorder
F06.7   Mild cognitive disorder
F06.8   Other specified mental disorders due to brain damage and dysfunction and to physical disease
F06.9   Unspecified mental disorder due to brain damage and dysfunction and to physical disease

F07   Personality and behavioural disorders due to brain disease, damage and dysfunction

F07.0   Organic personality disorder
F07.1   Postencephalitic syndrome
F07.2   Postconcussional syndrome
F07.8   Other organic personality and behavioural disorders due to brain disease, damage and dysfunction
F07.9   Unspecified organic personality and behavioural disorder due to brain disease, damage and dysfunction

F09   Unspecified organic or symptomatic mental disorder

F10–F19 Mental and behavioural disorders due to psychoactive substance use

F10   Mental and behavioural disorders due to use of alcohol
F11   Mental and behavioural disorders due to use of opioids
F12   Mental and behavioural disorders due to use of cannabinoids
F13   Mental and behavioural disorders due to use of sedatives or hypnotics
F14   Mental and behavioural disorders due to use of cocaine
F15   Mental and behavioural disorders due to use of other stimulants, including caffeine
F16   Mental and behavioural disorders due to use of hallucinogens
F17   Mental and behavioural disorders due to use of tobacco
F18   Mental and behavioural disorders due to use of volatile solvents

F19   Mental and behavioural disorders due to multiple drug use and use of other psychoactive substances

Four- and five-character categories may be used to specify the clinical conditions, as follows:

F1x.0   Acute intoxication:
.00   Uncomplicated
.01   With trauma or other bodily injury
.02   With other medical complications
.03   With delirium
.04   With perceptual distortions
.05   With coma
.06   With convulsions
.07   Pathological intoxication
F1x.1   Harmful use
Flx.2   Dependence syndrome:
.20   Currently abstinent
.21   Currently abstinent, but in a protected environment
.22   Currently on a clinically supervised maintenance or replacement regime (controlled dependence)
.23   Currently abstinent, but receiving treatment with aversive or blocking drugs
.24   Currently using the substance (active dependence)
.25   Continuous use
.26   Episodic use (dipsomania)
Flx.3   Withdrawal state:
.30   Uncomplicated
.31   With convulsions
Flx.4   Withdrawal state with delirium:
.40   Without convulsions
.41   With convulsions
F1x.5   Psychotic disorder:
.50   Schizophrenia-like
.51   Predominantly delusional
.52   Predominantly hallucinatory
.53   Predominantly polymorphic
.54   Predominantly depressive symptoms
.55   Predominantly manic symptoms
.56   Mixed
F1x.6   Amnesic syndrome
F1x.7   Residual and late-onset psychotic disorder:
.70   Flashbacks
.71   Personality or behaviour disorder
.72   Residual affective disorder
.73   Dementia

.74   Other persisting cognitive impairment
.75   Late-onset psychotic disorder
F1x.8 Other mental and behavioural disorders
F1x.9 Unspecified mental and behavioural disorder

F20–F29 Schizophrenia, schizotypal and delusional disorders
F20   Schizophrenia
F20.0 Paranoid schizophrenia
F20.1 Hebephrenic schizophrenia
F20.2 Catatonic schizophrenia
F20.3 Undifferentiated schizophrenia
F20.4 Postschizophrenic depression
F20.5 Residual schizophrenia
F20.6 Simple schizophrenia
F20.8 Other schizophrenia
F20.9 Schizophrenia, unspecified

A fifth character may be used to classify course:
.x0   Continuous
.xl   Episodic with progressive deficit
.x2   Episodic with stable deficit
.x3   Episodic remittent
.x4   Incomplete remission
.x5   Complete remission
.x8   Other
.x9   Course uncertain, period of observation too short

F21   Schizotypal disorder

F22   Persistent delusional disorders
F22.0 Delusional disorder
F22.8 Other persistent delusional disorders
F22.9 Persistent delusional disorder, unspecified

F23   Acute and transient psychotic disorders
F23.0 Acute polymorphic psychotic disorder without symptoms of schizophrenia
F23.1 Acute polymorphic psychotic disorder with symptoms of schizophrenia
F23.2 Acute schizophrenia-like psychotic disorder
F23.3 Other acute predominantly delusional psychotic disorders
F23.8 Other acute and transient psychotic disorders
F23.9 Acute and transient psychotic disorders unspecified

A fifth character may be used to identify the presence or absence of associated acute stress:

.;tO   Without associated acute stress

.x\   With associated acute stress

F24   Induced delusional disorder

F25   Schizoaffective disorders
F25.0   Schizoaffective disorder, manic type
F25.1   Schizoaffective disorder, depressive type
F25.2   Schizoaffective disorder, mixed type
F25.8   Other schizoaffective disorders
F25.9   Schizoaffective disorder, unspecified

F28   Other non-organic psychotic disorders

F29   Unspecified non-organic psychosis

F30–F39 Mood (affective) disorders
F30   Manic episode
F30.0   Hypomania
F30.1   Mania without psychotic symptoms
F30.2   Mania with psychotic symptoms
F30.8   Other manic episodes
F30.9   Manic episode, unspecified

F31   Bipolar affective disorder
F31.0   Bipolar affective disorder, current episode hypomanic
F31.1   Bipolar affective disorder, current episode manic without psychotic symptoms
F31.2   Bipolar affective disorder, current episode manic with psychotic symptoms
F31.3   Bipolar affective disorder, current episode mild or moderate depression:
.30   Without somatic syndrome
.31   With somatic syndrome
F31.4   Bipolar affective disorder, current episode severe depression without psychotic symptoms
F31.5   Bipolar affective disorder, current episode severe depression with psychotic symptoms
F31.6   Bipolar affective disorder, current episode mixed
F31.7   Bipolar affective disorder, currently in remission
F31.8   Other bipolar affective disorders
F31.9   Bipolar affective disorder, unspecified

F32 **Depressive episode**
F32.0 Mild depressive episode:
.00 Without somatic syndrome
.01 With somatic syndrome
F32.1 Moderate depressive episode:
.10 Without somatic syndrome
.11 With somatic syndrome
F32.2 Severe depressive episode without psychotic symptoms
F32.3 Severe depressive episode with psychotic symptoms
F32.8 Other depressive episodes
F32.9 Depressive episode, unspecified

F33 **Recurrent depressive disorder**
F33.0 Recurrent depressive disorder, current episode mild:
.00 Without somatic syndrome
.01 With somatic syndrome
F33.1 Recurrent depressive disorder, current episode moderate:
.10 Without somatic syndrome
.11 With somatic syndrome
F33.2 Recurrent depressive disorder, current episode severe without psychotic symptoms
F33.3 Recurrent depressive disorder, current episode severe with psychotic symptoms
F33.4 Recurrent depressive disorder, currently in remission
F33.8 Other recurrent depressive disorders
F33.9 Recurrent depressive disorder, unspecified

F34 **Persistent mood (affective) disorders**
F34.0 Cyclothymia
F34.1 Dysthymia
F34.8 Other persistent mood (affective) disorders
F34.9 Persistent mood (affective) disorder, unspecified

F38 **Other mood (affective) disorders**
F38.0 Other single mood (affective) disorders:
.00 Mixed affective episode
F38.1 Other recurrent mood (affective) disorders:
.10 Recurrent brief depressive disorder
F38.8 Other specified mood (affective) disorders

F39 **Unspecified mood (affective) disorder**

F40–F48 Neurotic, stress-related and somatoform disorders
F40 **Phobic anxiety disorders**
F40.0 Agoraphobia:

.00   Without panic disorder
.01   With panic disorder
F40.1   Social phobias
F40.2   Specific (isolated) phobias
F40.8   Other phobic anxiety disorders
F40.9   Phobic anxiety disorder, unspecified

F41   Other anxiety disorders
F41.0   Panic disorder (episodic paroxysmal anxiety)
F41.1   Generalised anxiety disorder
F41.2   Mixed anxiety and depressive disorder
F41.3   Other mixed anxiety disorders
F41.8   Other specified anxiety disorders
F41.9   Anxiety disorder, unspecified

F42   Obsessive-compulsive disorder
F42.0   Predominantly obsessional thoughts or ruminations
F42.1   Predominantly compulsive acts (obsessional rituals)
F42.2   Mixed obsessional thoughts and acts
F42.8   Other obsessive-compulsive disorders
F42.9   Obsessive-compulsive disorder, unspecified

F43   Reaction to severe stress, and adjustment disorders
F43.0   Acute stress reaction
F43.1   Post-traumatic stress disorder
F43.2   Adjustment disorders:
.20   Brief depressive reaction
.21   Prolonged depressive reaction
.22   Mixed anxiety and depressive reaction
.23   With predominant disturbance of other emotions
.24   With predominant disturbance of conduct
.25   With mixed disturbance of emotions and conduct
.28   With other specified predominant symptoms
F43.8   Other reactions to severe stress
F43.9   Reaction to severe stress, unspecified

F44   Dissociative (conversion) disorders
F44.0   Dissociative amnesia
F44.1   Dissociative fugue
F44.2   Dissociative stupor
F44.3   Trance and possession disorders
F44.4   Dissociative motor disorders
F44.5   Dissociative convulsions
F44.6   Dissociative anaesthesia and sensory loss
F44.7   Mixed dissociative (conversion) disorders

F44.8   Other dissociative (conversion) disorders:
.80   Ganser's syndrome
.81   Multiple personality disorder
.82   Transient dissociative (conversion) disorders occurring in childhood and adolescence
.88   Other specified dissociative (conversion) disorders
F44.9   Dissociative (conversion) disorder, unspecified

F45   Somatoform disorders
F45.0   Somatisation disorder
F45.1   Undifferentiated somatoform disorder
F45.2   Hypochondriacal disorder
F45.3   Somatoform autonomic dysfunction:
.30   Heart and cardiovascular system
.31   Upper gastrointestinal tract
.32   Lower gastrointestinal tract
.33   Respiratory system
.34   Genitourinary system
.38   Other organ or system
F45.4   Persistent somatoform pain disorder
F45.8   Other somatoform disorders
F45.9   Somatoform disorder, unspecified

F48   Other neurotic disorders
F48.0   Neurasthenia
F48.1   Depersonalisation-derealisation syndrome
F48.8   Other specified neurotic disorders
F48.9   Neurotic disorder, unspecified

F50–F59 Eating disorders
F50   Eating disorders
F50.0   Anorexia nervosa
F50.1   Atypical anorexia nervosa
F50.2   Bulimia nervosa
F50.3   Atypical bulimia nervosa
F50.4   Overeating associated with other psychological disturbances
F50.5   Vomiting associated with other psychological disturbances
F50.8   Other eating disorders
F50.9   Eating disorder, unspecified

F51   Non-organic sleep disorders
F51.0   Non-organic insomnia
F51.1   Non-organic hypersomnia
F51.2   Non-organic disorder of the sleep-wake schedule
F51.3   Sleepwalking (somnambulism)

F51.4 Sleep terrors (night terrors)
F51.5 Nightmares
F51.8 Other non-organic sleep disorders
F51.9 Non-organic sleep disorder, unspecified

F52 Sexual dysfunction, not caused by organic disorder or disease
F52.0 Lack or loss of sexual desire
F52.1 Sexual aversion and lack of sexual enjoyment:
.10   Sexual aversion
.11   Lack of sexual enjoyment
F52.2 Failure of genital response
F52.3 Orgasmic dysfunction
F52.4 Premature ejaculation
F52.5 Non-organic vaginismus
F52.6 Non-organic dyspareunia
F52.7 Excessive sexual drive
F52.8 Other sexual dysfunction, not caused by organic disorders or disease
F52.9 Unspecified sexual dysfunction, not caused by organic disorder or disease

F53 Mental and behavioural disorders associated with the puerperium, not elsewhere classified
F53.0 Mild mental and behavioural disorders associated with the puerperium, not elsewhere classified
F53.1 Severe mental and behavioural disorders associated with the puerperium, not elsewhere classified
F53.8 Other mental and behavioural disorders associated with the puerperium, not elsewhere classified
F53.9 Puerperal mental disorder, unspecified

F54 Psychological and behavioural factors associated with disorders or diseases classified elsewhere

F55 Abuse of non-dependence-producing substances
F55.0 Antidepressants
F55.1 Laxatives
F55.2 Analgesics
F55.3 Antacids
F55.4 Vitamins
F55.5 Steroids or hormones
F55.6 Specific herbal or folk remedies
F55.8 Other substances that do not produce dependence
F55.9 Unspecified

F59 **Unspecified behavioural syndromes associated with physiological disturbances and physical factors**

F60–F69 Personality disorders
F60 **Specific personality disorders**
F60.0 Paranoid personality disorder
F60.1 Schizoid personality disorder
F60.2 Dissocial personality disorder
F60.3 Emotionally unstable personality disorder:
.30 Impulsive type
.31 Borderline type
F60.4 Histrionic personality disorder
F60.5 Anankastic personality disorder
F60.6 Anxious (avoidant) personality disorder
F60.7 Dependent personality disorder
F60.8 Other specific personality disorders
F60.9 Personality disorder, unspecified

F61 **Mixed and other personality disorders**
F61.0 Mixed personality disorders
F61.1 Troublesome personality changes

F62 **Enduring personality changes, not attributable to brain damage and disease**
F62.0 Enduring personality change after catastrophic experience
F62.1 Enduring personality change after psychiatric illness
F62.8 Other enduring personality changes
F62.9 Enduring personality change, unspecified

F63 **Habit and impulse disorders**
F63.0 Pathological gambling
F63.1 Pathological fire-setting (pyromania)
F63.2 Pathological stealing (kleptomania)
F63.3 Trichotillomania
F63.8 Other habit and impulse disorders
F63.9 Habit and impulse disorder, unspecified

F64 **Gender identity disorders**
F64.0 Transsexualism
F64.1 Dual-role transvestism
F64.2 Gender identity disorder of childhood
F64.8 Other gender identity disorders
F64.9 Gender identity disorder, unspecified

F65   Disorders of sexual preference

F65.0   Fetishism
F65.1   Fetishistic transvestism
F65.2   Exhibitionism
F65.3   Voyeurism
F65.4   Paedophilia
F65.5   Sadomasochism
F65.6   Multiple disorders of sexual preference
F65.8   Other disorders of sexual preference
F65.9   Disorder of sexual preference, unspecified

F66   Psychological and behavioural disorders associated with sexual development and orientation

F66.0   Sexual maturation disorder
F66.1   Egodystonic sexual orientation
F66.2   Sexual relationship disorder
F66.8   Other psychosexual development disorders
F66.9   Psychosexual development disorder, unspecified

F68   Other disorders of adult personality and behaviour

F68.0   Elaboration of physical symptoms for psychological reasons
F68.1   Intentional production or feigning of symptoms or disabilities, either physical or psychological (factitious disorder)
F68.8   Other specified disorders of adult personality and behaviour

F69   Unspecified disorder of adult personality and behaviour

F70–F79 Learning disability
F70   Mild mental retardation
F71   Moderate mental retardation
F72   Severe mental retardation
F73   Profound mental retardation
F78   Other mental retardation
F79   Unspecified mental retardation

A fourth character may be used to specify the extent of associated behavioural impairment:

F1x.0   No, or minimal, impairment of behaviour
Flx.1   Significant impairment of behaviour requiring attention or treatment
F1x.8   Other impairments of behaviour
F1x.9   Without mention of impairment of behaviour

F80–F89 Psychological development disorders
F80   Specific developmental disorders of speech and language
F80.0   Specific speech articulation disorder
F80.1   Expressive language disorder
F80.2   Receptive language disorder
F80.3   Acquired aphasia with epilepsy (Landau–Kieffner syndrome)
F80.8   Other developmental disorders of speech and language
F80.9   Developmental disorder of speech and language, unspecified

F81   Specific developmental disorders of scholastic skills
F81.0   Specific reading disorder
F81.1   Specific spelling disorder
F81.2   Specific disorder of arithmetical skills
F81.3   Mixed disorder of scholastic skills
F81.8   Other developmental disorders of scholastic skills
F81.9   Developmental disorder of scholastic skills, unspecified

F82   Specific developmental disorder of motor function

F83   Mixed specific developmental disorders

F84   Pervasive developmental disorders
F84.0   Childhood autism
F84.1   Atypical autism
F84.2   Rett's syndrome
F84.3   Other childhood disintegrative disorder
F84.4   Overactive disorder associated with mental retardation and stereotyped movements
F84.5   Asperger's syndrome
F84.8   Other pervasive developmental disorders
F84.9   Pervasive developmental disorder, unspecified

F88   Other disorders of psychological development

F89   Unspecified disorder of psychological development

F90–F98 Childhood and adolescence
F90   Hyperkinetic disorders
F90.0   Disturbance of activity and attention
F90.1   Hyperkinetic conduct disorder
F90.8   Other hyperkinetic disorders
F90.9   Hyperkinetic disorder, unspecified

F91   Conduct disorders
F91.0   Conduct disorder confined to the family context

F91.1   Unsocialised conduct disorder
F91.2   Socialised conduct disorder
F91.3   Oppositional defiant disorder
F91.8   Other conduct disorders
F91.9   Conduct disorder, unspecified

F92   Mixed disorders of conduct and emotions
F92.0   Depressive conduct disorder
F92.8   Other mixed disorders of conduct and emotions
F92.9   Mixed disorder of conduct and emotions, unspecified

F93   Emotional disorders with onset specific to childhood
F93.0   Separation anxiety disorder of childhood
F93.1   Phobic anxiety disorder of childhood
F93.2   Social anxiety disorder of childhood
F93.3   Sibling rivalry disorder
F93.8   Other childhood emotional disorders
F93.9   Childhood emotional disorder, unspecified

F94   Disorders of social functioning with onset specific to childhood and adolescence
F94.0   Elective mutism
F94.1   Reactive attachment disorder of childhood
F94.2   Disinhibited attachment disorder of childhood
F94.8   Other childhood disorders of social functioning
F94.9   Childhood disorders of social functioning, unspecified

F95   Tic disorders
F95.0   Transient tic disorder
F95.1   Chronic motor or vocal tic disorder
F95.2   Combined vocal and multiple motor tic disorder (de la Tourette's syndrome)
F95.8   Other tic disorders
F95.9   Tic disorder, unspecified

F98   Other behavioural and emotional disorders with onset usually occurring in childhood and adolescence
F98.0   Non-organic enuresis
F98.1   Non-organic encopresis
F98.2   Feeding disorder of infancy and childhood
F98.3   Pica of infancy and childhood
F98.4   Stereotyped movement disorders
F98.5   Stuttering (stammering)
F98.6   Cluttering

F98.8   Other specified behavioural and emotional disorders with onset usually occurring in childhood and adolescence

F98.9   Unspecified behavioural and emotional disorders with onset usually occurring in childhood and adolescence

F99 Mental disorder, not otherwise specified

All others not fitting any other category are covered here

Chapter 1

Organic mental disorders (F00–F09)

General criteria for dementia (G1–G4)

G1 **M**emory decline– especially for new information (mild/moderate/severe)
Thinking and judgement deterioration (mild/moderate/severe) – objective evidence is required
G2 **A**bsence of clouding of consciousness
G3 **E**motional control decline: *L*ability, *I*rritability, *A*pathy and *B*ehavioural changes (*BAIL*)
G4 G1 present for at least **S**ix months – for confidence

Memory deficit for new information
Absence of clouding of consciousness
Thinking and judgement deficit
Emotional control decline (*BAIL*)
Six months duration (at least)

MATES

'Lots of social support (in the form of "good mates") is required in dementia'

F00 Dementia in Alzheimer's disease

1. General (G1–G4) criteria for dementia are met
2. No evidence for any other causes for the dementia (e.g. HIV, reversible causes of dementia, etc.)

The diagnosis is ultimately confirmed by postmortem evidence

F00.0 Dementia in Alzheimer's disease with early onset
1. Criteria for F00 met, and age of onset should be below 65 years
2. One of the following met:
   i. Rapid onset and progression
   ii. In addition to memory impairment, must be *aphasia, agraphia, alexia, acalculia* or *apraxia* (5As – signs of cortical dysfunction)

Dementia general criteria (F00) met
Rapid onset and progression
Age – younger (<65 years)
Multiple disorders of cortical function + memory affected
A 5As – *aphasia, agraphia, alexia, acalculia or apraxia*

DRAMA

F00.1 Dementia in Alzheimer's disease with late onset
Late onset, i.e. >65 years
1. Criteria for F00 met
2. One of the following:
   i. Slow onset and progression (*usually identified after 3 years or more*)
   ii. Predominance of a memory impairment, over intellectual impairment

Slow onset and progression
Age – late onset (>65 years old)
Memory impairment

SAM

F00.2 Dementia in Alzheimer's disease, atypical or mixed type
Atypical dementias
Mixed vascular and Alzheimer's dementia are included in this category

F00.9 Dementia in Alzheimer's disease, unspecified

F01 Vascular dementia

This is usually a later-onset dementia (i.e. >65 years old), which is infarct induced. It is as a result of brain tissue infarction due to vascular disease

G1 General criteria for dementia G1–G4 met
G2 Unevenly distributed deficits in higher cognitive function deficits, with some functions affected and others relatively spared
G3 Clinical evidence of focal brain damage (shown by at least one of the following):
   1. unilaterally increased tendon reflexes *R*
   2. an extensor plantar response *E*
   3. pseudobulbar palsy *P*
   4. unilateral spastic weakness of the limbs *S* (*REPS*)
G4 There is evidence from the history, examination or tests of significant cerebrovascular disease

Clinical evidence (*REPS*)
of focal brain damage
Unevenly distributed deficits in higher cognitive function
General criteria for dementia met
History and examination suggestive of cerebrovascular disease

CoUGH

F01.0 Vascular dementia of acute onset
A. Criteria for F01 met (**CoUGH**)
B. Dementia develops *rapidly*, i.e. usually within one month (*but not longer than three months*) after a succession of strokes or after a single infarct

F01.1 Multi-infarct dementia
Usually a cortical dementia:
A. Criteria for F01 met (**CoUGH**)
B. Onset is *gradual* within 3–6 months following a number of minor ischaemic episodes
Thought to be as a result of an *accumulation* of infarcts in the brain matter. There may be some possible *improvement between ischaemic episodes*

F01.2 Subcortical vascular dementia

A. Criteria for F01 met (**CoUGH**)
B. Hypertension history
C. Clinical examination and investigations show vascular disease in the deep white matter of the cerebral hemispheres, with *preservation* of the cerebral cortex

Hypertension history
Investigation displays evidence of vascular disease in the deep white matter
Preservation of the cerebral cortex

HIP

F01.3 Mixed cortical and subcortical vascular dementia
Evidence of both of the above via investigations

F01.8 Other vascular dementia

F01.9 Vascular dementia unspecified

F02 Dementia in other diseases classified elsewhere

F02.0 Dementia in Pick's disease

A. General criteria for dementia (G1–G4) met
B. Onset is slow and displays a steady deterioration
C. Predominance of frontal lobe involvement *(two of the following)*: *a*phasia, *a*pathy, *b*lunting of emotions, *c*oarsening of social behaviour, *d*isinhibition (A_2BCD)
D. In early stages, memory and parietal lobe functions are relatively preserved

Frontal (A_2BCD)
Onset slow
General criteria

FOG

F02.1 Dementia in Creutzfeldt–Jakob disease (CJD)

A. General criteria for dementia (G1–G4) met
B. Rapid progression with disintegration of virtually all higher cerebral function
C. 1/ more:
  1. *P*yramidal symptoms
  2. *E*xtrapyramidal symptoms
  3. *A*phasia
  4. *C*erebellar symptoms
  5. *E*ye/visual impairment (*PEACE*)

Akinetic and mute stage is usually the typical terminal stage
Amyotrophic variant seen
Characteristic electroencephalograph (EEG)
Diagnosis only confirmed by neuropathological examination

Terminal akinetic stage
Amyotrophic variant
Pathological examination confirms diagnosis
EEG demonstrates a characteristic pattern

TAPE + PEACE

F02.2 Dementia in Huntington's disease
A. General criteria for dementia (G1–G4) met
B. Subcortical functions affected first – *S*lowness of thinking, or *M*ovement and *P*ersonality alteration, with *A*pathy or *D*epression (*DAMPS*)
C. Involuntary choreiform movements
D. Family history of Huntington's disease
E. No clinical features that account for the abnormal movements

*S*ubcortical (*DAMPS*) functions affected first
*C*horeiform movements
A clear family history
*N*o clinical features to account for the abnormal movements

SCAN

F02.3 Dementia in Parkinson's disease
A. General criteria for dementia (G1–G4) met
B. Diagnosis of Parkinson's disease has been established
C. None of the cognitive impairment is attributable to anti-parkinsonian medication
D. No evidence of other forms of dementia, brain disease, systemic disorder or alcohol or drug abuse

*P*arkinson disease has been established
*A*nti-parkinson medications unrelated
*N*o evidence of other forms of dementia or other disease

PAN

F02.4 Dementia in HIV disease
A. General criteria for dementia (G1–G4) met
B. Diagnosis of HIV infection has been established
C. No evidence of other forms of dementia, brain disease, systemic disorder or alcohol or drug abuse

*D*ementia general criteria met
*E*stablished diagnosis of HIV
*N*o evidence of any other potential causes

DEN

F02.8 Dementia in other specified diseases classified elsewhere
Dementia occurring as a consequence of a variety of cerebral and somatic conditions, which are classified in other chapters of ICD-10

F03 Unspecified dementia

General criteria fulfilled but it is not possible to identify one of the specific types

F04 Organic amnesic syndrome, not induced by alcohol and other psychoactive substances

Impairment of *R*ecent and *R*emote memory whilst *I*mmediate recall is preserved (*R+R > I*)
Reduced ability to *learn new material* and *disorientation* in time
Confabulation may be prominent but perception and other cognitive functions are unaffected
The prognosis is dependent on the underlying lesion

A. Memory impairment is seen in:
    i.   Recent memory (impaired learning of new material)
    ii. Ability to recall past experiences
B. Absence of:
    i.   Defect in immediate recall (e.g. via digit span test)
    ii. Clouding of consciousness and attention disturbance
    iii. Global intellectual decline (dementia)
C. Objective evidence of a disease of the brain (i.e. through clinical history, examination and investigations)

Clouding of consciousness is *absent*
Objective evidence present of a disease of the brain
Past experiences are hard to recall
Immediate recall relatively preserved, but remote + recent impaired
New material learning is impaired
Global intellectual decline is absent

COPING

F05 Delirium, not induced by alcohol and other psychoactive substances

A. Clouding of consciousness (loss of clear awareness of the environment and reduced ability to focus and maintain attention)
B. Cognition disturbance:
   i. Reduced immediate and recent recall, with relatively intact remote memory
   ii. Disorientation in time/place/person
C. Psychomotor disturbances: 1/more of the following:
   i. Hypo/hyperactivity shifts
   ii. Increased reaction time
   iii. Increased/decreased flow of speech
   iv. Enhanced startle reaction
D. Sleep-wake cycle or sleep disturbance: 1/more of the following:
   i. Insomnia +/- daytime drowsiness or reversal of the sleep-wake cycle
   ii. Nocturnal worsening of symptoms
   iii. Disturbing dreams and nightmares
E. Rapid onset with fluctuating symptoms over the course of the day
F. Objective evidence of an underlying cerebral or systemic disease responsible for the clinical manifestations

Cognition disturbance
Objective evidence of underlying disease
Rapid onset
Psychomotor disturbance
Sleep-wake cycle disturbance
Everything is clouded (clouded consciousness)

CORPSE

F05.0 Delirium not superimposed on dementia

F05.1 Delirium superimposed on dementia

F05.8 Other delirium
Delirium of mixed origin

F05.9 Delirium, unspecified

F06 Other mental disorders due to brain damage and dysfunction and to physical disease

Includes miscellaneous conditions causally related to brain disorder due to primary cerebral disease, or conditions affecting the brain secondarily

G1 Objective evidence present of cerebral disease, or other cause known to cause cerebral dysfunction

G2 There is a presumed relationship of the underlying disease/disorder/dysfunction and the mental disorder

G3 Recovery from the mental disorder following the removal or improvement of the presumed underlying cause

G4 Insufficient evidence for an alternative causation of the mental disorder

Relationship of the disease and the mental disorder is presumed
Objective evidence present of cerebral disease
Alternative cause unlikely
Recovery from the mental disorder after removal of the underlying cause

ROAR

F06.0 Organic hallucinosis

A disorder of persistent or recurrent hallucinations: usually visual or auditory, occurring in clear consciousness. Delusional elaboration of the hallucinations may occur but delusions do not dominate the clinical picture. Insight may or may not be present

A. General criteria for F06 met
B. Dominated by persistent hallucinations (usually visual or auditory)
C. Hallucinations occur in clear consciousness

Clear consciousness hallucinations
All of the general criteria for F06 met
Persistent hallucinations present

CAP

F06.1 Organic catatonic disorder
A disorder of reduced (stupor) or increased (excitement) of psychomotor activity associated with catatonic symptoms

A. General criteria for F06 met
B. One of the following must be present:
    i. Stupor (a diminution or absence of voluntary movements and speech with normal responsiveness to light, noise and touch with positive resistance to passive movement of limbs)
    ii. Negativism (resistance to passive movement of limbs or body with rigid posturing)
C. Catatonic excitement (extreme hypermotility)
D. Rapid alternation between stupor and excitement

Catatonic excitement
Alternation between stupor and excitement
Negativism
Stupor

CANS

Diagnostic confidence increased if additional catatonic phenomena are present and care should be made to exclude delirium

F06.2 Organic delusional (schizophrenia-like) disorder
Some features of schizophrenia, such as bizarre hallucinations and thought disorders, may be present. Recurrent delusions dominate the clinical picture. The delusions may be present with hallucinations

A. General criteria for F06 must be met
B. Clinical picture dominated by delusions (e.g. persecution/bodily change/disease/death/jealousy) which may show varying degrees of systemisation
C. Consciousness is clear and memory is intact

Clear consciousness
Delusions with varying levels of systematisation

CD

Includes paranoid-hallucinatory organic states, and schizophrenia-like psychosis in epilepsy

F06.3 Organic mood (affective) disorders
A. General criteria for F06 must be met
B. Meets the criteria for <u>one of the affective disorders</u>, i.e. manic, bipolar, depressive, mixed affective disorder (F30–F32)

F06.4 Organic anxiety disorder
A. General criteria for F06 must be met
B. The condition must meet the criteria for <u>either</u> F41.0 (Panic Disorder) <u>or</u> F41.1 (Generalised Anxiety Disorder (GAD))

F06.5 Organic dissociative disorder
Loss of normal integration (partial/complete) between: *P*ast memories/*R*ecall, *I*dentity awareness and immediate *S*ensations and control of bodily *M*ovements (*PRISM*)

A. General criteria for F06 must be met
B. The condition must meet the criteria for F44.0–F44.8

F06.6 Organic emotionally labile (asthenic) disorder
A. General criteria for F06 met
B. Dominated by emotional lability (uncontrolled expression of emotion)
C. Variety of unpleasant physical sensations, i.e. dizziness and aches and pains

Criteria for F06 must be met
Unpleasant physical sensations
Emotional lability

CUE

F06.7 Mild cognitive impairment
A. General criteria for F06 met
B. Disorder in cognitive function most of the time over a period of at least two weeks. Any of the following:
   i. Memory (especially recall) or new learning
   ii. Attention/concentration
   iii. Thinking
   iv. Language
   v. Visuo-spatial functioning – *M*emory, *E*verything *N*ot seen (visuo-spatial), *T*hinking, *A*ttention, *L*anguage (*MENTAL*)
C. Abnormality in performance in quantified cognitive assessments
D. Excludes dementia/psychoactive related/delirium/organic amnesic/ postencephalitic/postconcussional syndrome

General criteria for F06 met
Assessment performance poor
Two-week (minimum) history of cognitive impairment (*MENTAL*)
Excludes others

GATE

F06.8 Other specified mental disorders due to brain damage and dysfunction and to physical disease
Examples include transient mild abnormal mood states occurring with treatment with antidepressants or steroids or epileptic psychosis not otherwise specified (NOS)

F06.9 Unspecified mental disorder due to brain damage and dysfunction and to physical disease
Organic brain syndrome and mental disorder NOS

F07 Disorders of personality and behaviour due to brain disease, damage and dysfunction

G1 Objective evidence of brain disease, damage or dysfunction
G2 No clouding of consciousness or significant memory deficit
G3 There is insufficient evidence of a personality or behavioural disorder justifying F60–F69

Exclusions should be noted (F60–F69)
Clouding of consciousness absent
Objective evidence of brain disease, damage or dysfunction

ECO

Note: 'Think organic ecosystem'

F07.0 Organic personality disorder
A. F07 general criteria met
B. Three or more of the following over a period of six months:
    i.   Reduced ability to persevere in goal-related activities
    ii. Emotional changes
    iii. Disinhibited expression of needs
    iv. Cognitive and attention disturbances
    v. Alteration of rate and flow of language production

Goal-related activities reduced
Language production altered
Attention/cognitive disturbances
Disinhibition
Emotional changes
Six months

GLADES

Note: Different personality disorder subtypes that can be ascribed to this diagnosis

F07.1 Postencephalitic syndrome

This is a residual non-specific/variable behavioural change following recovery from either viral or bacterial encephalitis. Compared to F07.0, it is reversible

A. General criteria for F07 met
B. 1/-:
    i. *A*phasia
    ii. *P*aralysis
    iii. *A*calculia
    iv. *C*onstructional apraxia
    v. *H*earing loss/deafness (*APACH*)
C. The syndrome is *reversible* and its duration rarely Exceeds 24 months

APACH (as above) + **E**xceeds 24 months very rarely

APACHE

F07.2 Postconcussional syndrome

This is a syndrome that can occur following head trauma (usually) severe enough to induce a loss of consciousness

A. General criteria for F07 met
B. There must be a history of head trauma with loss of consciousness preceding the onset of symptoms by a period of up to four weeks (objective investigations/imaging may be lacking)
C. At least three of:
    i. Complaints of unpleasant sensations and pains: headaches, dizziness, general malaise and excessive fatigue or noise sensitivity
    ii. Emotional changes – irritability and emotional lability or some degree of depression or anxiety
    iii. Subjective complaints of difficulty in concentration and in performing mental tasks and of memory problems (without clear objective evidence)
    iv. Insomnia
    v. Reduced tolerance to alcohol
    vi. Preoccupation of the above symptoms and fear of permanent brain damage, to the extent of hypochondriacal overvalued ideas and adoption of a sick role

Emotional changes
Tolerance reduced to alcohol
Hypochondriachal + head trauma
Insomnia
Concentration subjectively reduced
Sensation alteration

ETHICS

F07.8 Other organic personality and behavioural disorders due to brain disease, damage and dysfunction
Disorders that are not classifiable elsewhere

F07.9 Unspecified organic personality and behavioural disorders due to brain disease, damage and dysfunction
Organic psychosyndrome

F09 Unspecified organic or symptomatic mental disorder

Other mental disorders derived from an organic aetiology

Summary

General criteria for dementia
MATES

F00.0 Dementia in Alzheimer's disease with early onset
DRAMA

F00.1 Dementia in Alzheimer's disease with late onset
SAM

F01 Vascular dementia
CoUGH

F01.2 Subcortical vascular dementia
HIP

F02.0 Dementia in Pick's disease
FOG

F02.1 Dementia in CJD
PEACE TAPE

F02.2 Dementia in Huntington's disease
SCAN

F02. 3 Dementia in Parkinson's disease
PAN

F02.4 Dementia in HIV disease
DEN

F04 Organic amnesic syndrome, not induced by alcohol and other psychoactive substances
COPING

F05 Delirium, not induced by alcohol and other psychoactive substances
CORPSE

F06 Other mental disorders due to brain damage and dysfunction and to physical disease
ROAR

F06.0 Organic hallucinosis
CAP

F06.1 Organic catatonic disorder
CANS

F06.2 Organic delusional disorder (schizophrenia like)
CD

F06.5 Organic dissociative disorder
PRISM

F06.6 Organic emotionally unstable (asthenic) disorder
CUE

F06.7 Mild cognitive impairment
GATE

F07 Personality and behavioural disorders due to brain disease, damage and dysfunction
ECO

F07.0 Organic personality disorder
GLADES

F07.1 Postencephalitic syndrome
APACHE

F07.2 Postconcussional syndrome
ETHICS

Chapter 2

Mental and behavioural disorders due to psychoactive substance use (F10–F19)

Stimulant (F15.-)
Sedative (F13.-)
Solvents (volatile) (F18.-)
Tobacco (F17.-)
Opioids (F11.-)
Multiple psychoactive substance use (F19.-)
Alcohol (F10.-)
Cannabinoids (F12.-)
Cocaine (F14.-)
Hallucinogens (F16.-)

S₃TOMAC₂H

F1x.0 Acute intoxication
A. Clear Evidence of recent use of a psychoactive substance
B. Symptoms or signs of intoxication Compatible with the known actions of the particular substances, producing disturbances in consciousness, perception, affect or behaviour
C. Symptoms or signs are not Accounted for by a medical disorder or by another mental and behavioural disorder
This is used for specific substances, e.g. F10.0 – alcohol and F11.0 – opioids

Another mental and behavioural disorder does not account for the symptoms/signs
Compatible with known actions of substances
Evidence of recent use

ACE

Flx.1 Harmful use
A. Clear Evidence that the substance use was responsible/contributed to physical or psychological harm including impaired judgment or dysfunctional behaviour
B. The Nature of the harm should be clearly identified and specified
C. The pattern of use has occurred for at least one month or has occurred repeatedly within a 12-month period – Duration
D. Does not meet the criteria for any other mental or behavioural disorder related to the same drug in the same time period (except acute intoxication Flx.0)

Evidence that substance use is responsible for harm
Nature of harm clearly identified
Duration occurred for at least one month or has occurred repeatedly within a 12-month period

END

Flx.2 Dependence syndrome
A. 3/- more of (over at least one month or if <1 month, repeatedly within a 12-month period):
    i. Compulsion to take the substance
    ii. Withdrawal state when the substance is reduced or stopped (physiological)
    iii. Reinstatement after abstinence or problems controlling behaviours
    iv. Incessant use despite evidence of harmful consequences
    v. Salience over other activities
    vi. Tolerance to the effects of the substance

C-WRIST

Note: For example, alcohol dependence is a risk factor for a Colles' wrist fracture

Further subtyping: describing its use and course

F1x.3 Withdrawal state
G1 Clear evidence of recent cessation/reduction
G2 Symptoms or signs compatible with known features of a withdrawal state from the particular substance(s)
G3 Symptoms or signs are not accounted for by a medical disorder or by another mental and behavioural disorder

Compatible with known features of a withdrawal state
Another mental and behavioural disorder does not account for the symptoms or signs
Recent cessation or reduction of the substance

CAR

F1x.4 Withdrawal with delirium
A. General criteria for Withdrawal
B. General criteria for Delirium met
+/- Convulsions (a further subdivision – F1x.40 without convulsions and F1x.41 with convulsions)

Withdrawal
and
Delirium

WaD

F1x.5 Psychotic disorder
A. Onset of psychotic symptoms must occur during/within two weeks of the substance use
B. Psychotic symptoms persist for >48 hours
C. Duration does not exceed six months
Note: The different subtypes of this disorder

Persists for >48 hours
Onset is within two weeks of the substance use
Duration <6 months

POD

F1x.6 Amnesic syndrome

A. Memory impairment in both:
- i. defective recent memory (especially learning new material)
- ii. reduced ability to recall past experiences

B. All of the following are absent:
- i. defective immediate recall
- ii. clouding of consciousness and disturbance of attention
- iii. global intellectual decline (i.e. dementia)

C. No objective evidence that any other conditions could be responsible for the clinical manifestations in A

Recent + recall for past memory display chronic impairment
Immediate recall is preserved
Confabulation may be present, clouding of consciousness and other cognitive deficits usually absent
Exclude any other disorders that could be present

RICE

F1x.7 Residual and late-onset psychotic disorder
Psychoactive-induced changes persist beyond the period during which a direct substance-related effect would be assumed to be operating

A. Conditions meeting individual syndromes (below) that should be linked to substance use

B. A fifth character is used:
- i. Flashbacks (F1x.70)
- ii. Personality or behaviour disorder (F1x.71)
- iii. Residual affective disorder (F1x.72)
- iv. Dementia (F1x.73)
- v. Other persisting cognitive impairment (F1x.74)
- vi. Late-onset psychotic disorder (F1x.75)

Affective (residual) disorder
Behavioural and personality
Cognitive (other)
Dementia
'**E**leventh hour'/late-onset psychotic disorder
Flashbacks

ABCDEF

F1x.8 Other mental and behavioural disorder

F1x.9 Unspecified mental and behavioural disorders

Summary

S_3TOMAC_2H

F1x.0 Acute intoxication
ACE

F1x.1 Harmful use
END

F1x.2 Dependence syndrome
C-WRIST

F1x.3 Withdrawal state
CAR

F1x.4 Withdrawal with delirium
WaD

F1x.5 Psychotic disorder
POD

F1x.6 Amnesic syndrome
RICE

F1x.7 Residual and late-onset psychotic disorder
ABCDEF

Chapter 3

Schizophrenia, schizotypal and delusional disorders (F20–F29)

F20 General criteria

Symptoms present for at least a month's duration
In schizophrenia: '*CDs and TVs create a NICHE*'
Associated with ideas of reference (audio (CDs) and visual (TVs))

<u>EITHER:</u>
G1 1.a–d
At least 1/- of:
a. Control – delusions of control/influence/passivity referred to body/limb movements or specific thoughts, actions or sensations and delusional perception
b. Delusions – persistent, culturally inappropriate and impossible
c. Thoughts – echo/withdrawal/insertion/broadcasting
d. Voices – hallucinatory: running commentary, discussing the individual or other voices coming from some part of the body

<u>OR:</u>
G1 2. a–d
At least 2/- of:
a. Negative symptoms – apathy, paucity of speech + blunting/incongruity of affect
b. Incoherence – irrelevant speech: neologisms, breaks/interpolations in train of thought
c. Catatonic behaviour – waxy flexibility, excitement, posturing, mutism and stupor

d. Hallucinations – persistent in any modality occurring every day for at least one month

G2
Exclusions:
1. Affective disorder
2. Organic brain disease
3. Psychoactive substance related
'*CDs* and *TVs create a NICHE*'

F20.0 Paranoid schizophrenia
Paranoid schizophrenia is one of the most common types of schizophrenia

A. General criteria for F20 are met
B. Positive symptoms – prominent delusions or hallucinations (for example, reference, exalted birth, special mission, persecution, bodily change, jealousy, etc.)
C. Flattening or incongruity of affect/catatonic symptoms/incoherent speech can be present but *must not dominate* the clinical picture

General criteria for F20 are met
Affect changes can be present
Positive symptoms predominate

GAP

F20.1 Hebephrenic schizophrenia
Normally diagnosed only in children and young adults
Usually carries a poor prognosis

A. General criteria for F20 are met
B. **A**ffect changes:
    i. Definite and sustained flattening or shallowness of affect; or
    ii. Definite and sustained incongruity or inappropriateness of affect
C. Either:
    i. **B**ehaviour changes; or
    ii. **C**oherence of thoughts – definite thought disorder, speech is disjointed or incoherent
D. **D**elusions/hallucinations do not dominate the clinical picture

Affect changes
Behavioural changes/Coherence of thoughts
Delusions and hallucinations not dominating the clinical picture

A(B/C)D

F20.2 Catatonic schizophrenia
General criteria for F20 are met and *other possible causes of catatonic behaviours have been excluded*
Occurs for a period of at least two weeks
One or more of the following catatonic behaviours:

Stupor (marked decrease in reactivity)/mutism
Posturing (voluntary assumption + maintenance of odd postures)
Automatism to commands (automatic compliance with instructions)
Waxy flexibility (maintenance of limbs/body in imposed positions)
Negativism (motiveless resistance to all attempts to be moved)
Excitement (purposeless motor activity)
Rigidity (maintenance of a rigid posture)

SPAWNER

F20.3 Undifferentiated schizophrenia
General criteria for F20 are met
Insufficient symptoms to meet the criteria for any of the other subtypes

OR:
So many symptoms that more than one subtype is met

F20.4 Post-schizophrenic depression
This is a depressive episode after a episode of schizophrenia
The symptoms of schizophrenia do not dominate the clinical presentation
Episodes are frequently associated with an increased suicide risk

General criteria for schizophrenia (F20) met within the previous 12 months
One of the G1 2. a–d criteria (*see above at F20*)
The depressive symptoms must fulfil the criteria for *At Least* a *mild depressive episode*

GOAL

'One of the goals of effective management for schizophrenia is being aware of post-schizophrenic depression, due to the risk of suicide'

F20.5 Residual schizophrenia

A chronic stage in a schizophrenic illness characterised by prominent 'negative' symptoms

General criteria for F20 are met in the past
At least 4/- of the following over the past 12 months:

Reduction in psychomotor activity
Enterprise/initiative reduced
Affect blunted
Social performance poor/**S**elf-care poor
Oral output reduced – speech poverty
Non-verbal communication is poor

REAS$_2$ON

F20.6 Simple schizophrenia

**Personal behaviour deterioration
No **E**vidence of G1 symptoms or positive symptoms or organic brain disease
**Negative symptoms (apathy, underactivity, paucity of speech, blunting of affect, passivity, lack of initiative and poor non-verbal communication)
**Social performance decline
Slow progressive development over *at least one year*

* All three must be present

PENS

F20.8 Other schizophrenia

F20.9 Unspecified schizophrenia

F21 Schizotypal disorder

This comes under schizophrenia due to its relationship that separates it from a personality disorder The disorder does not meet the criteria for schizophrenia

At least *two years'* duration of *four or more* of the following:

Rapport – poor socially
Affect – inappropriate/constricted
Perceptual experiences – bodily, illusions, depersonalisation or derealisation
Paranoid/suspicious ideas
Odd beliefs/magical thinking
Odd/eccentric behaviour
Ruminations often without inner resistance
Transient pseudo-psychotic symptoms
Thinking stereotyped/vague/circumstantial

RAPPO$_2$RT$_2$

F22 Persistent delusional disorders

A variety of disorders in which long-standing delusions are the main characteristic

F22.0 Delusional disorder

A **DE**lusion or set of related delusions, other than those listed in F20
Lasts at least three months
Unfulfilled F20-F20.3 (general schizophrenia) criteria
Depressive symptoms can be present intermittently
Exclusions – organic mental disorder, or psychotic disorder due to psychoactive substance use, or persistent hallucinations excluded

DELUDE

Various types: persecutory/litigious/self-referential/grandiose/ hypochondriachal/jealous/erotomanic

F22.8 Other persistent delusional disorders

This is a category of persistent delusional disorder that does not meet the criteria for delusional disorder (F22.0) or schizophrenia (F20). This category is used when the delusion(s) are accompanied by schizophrenic symptoms that are insufficient to justify a diagnosis of F20

F22.9 Persistent delusional disorder, unspecified

F23 Acute and transient psychotic disorders

G1 **A**cute onset of symptoms – does not exceed two weeks
G2 **C**louding of consciousness is absent
G3 **U**nipolar/bipolar (affective disorder) criteria unmet
G4 **T**oxic substance-induced disorders are excluded
G5 **E**xclusion criteria – organic mental disorder or serious metabolic disturbances

ACUTE

F23.0 Acute polymorphic disorder without symptoms of schizophrenia
A. General criteria for F23 are met (**ACUTE**)
B. **R**apid symptom change: from day to day or within the same day
C. **H**allucination (any) or delusions: **P**ositive psychotic symptoms
D. **S**ymptoms: two of *Perplexity, Affect turmoil, Motility (PAM)*
E. If any symptoms listed for schizophrenia are present, they are only present for the *minority* of time
F. **D**uration *does not* exceed three months

Rapid symptom change
ACUTE (general criteria for F23 met)
Positive psychotic symptoms
If any symptoms listed for F20 are present, they are present for a short time
Duration (does not exceed three months)
Symptoms (*PAM*)

RAPIDS

F23.1 Acute polymorphic disorder with symptoms of schizophrenia
A. Criteria **A-D** of acute polymorphic disorder (F23.0) met
B. *Some* of the symptoms for **S**chizophrenia must have been present for the *majority of time* since the onset. The full criteria do not need to be met for (F20.-)
C. Symptoms in B *do not persist* >1 month (**D**uration)

A-D criteria of F23.0 met
Duration does not persist more than a month
Some symptoms for **S**chizophrenia, present for the majority of time

A-DDS

F23.2 Acute schizophrenia-like psychotic disorder
A. General criteria for F23 met
B. Criteria for schizophrenia met except the criterion for *duration*
C. Criteria B,C,D for F23.0 unmet
D. Total duration does not exceed one month

F23.3 Other acute predominantly delusional psychotic disorders
A. General criteria for F23 met
B. Stable delusions and hallucinations are present but do not fulfil F20–F20.3
C. Does not meet criteria for F23.0
D. Total duration is less than three months

F23.8 Other acute and transient psychotic disorders

F23.9 Acute and transient psychotic disorder, unspecified
Includes reactive psychosis and brief reactive psychosis, NOS

F24 Induced delusional disorder

A. An individual develops a delusion/delusional system held by someone else with a disorder in F20–23
B. The people concerned have an unusually close relationship with one another and are relatively isolated from others
C. Individuals must not have held the relevant belief before contact with the other person and must not have suffered from any other disorder classified in F20–23

Isolated individuals
Not suffering from other disorders
Develop a delusional system
Unusually close relationship between the people
Contact induced
Excluded, **D**isorders: F20–23

INDUCED

F25 Schizoaffective disorders

Both affective + psychotic symptoms are present together
Mixed, manic and depressive subtypes

G1 Criteria for one **A**ffective disorder met (F30 – F31 – F32)
G2 Symptoms – *one or more* – for at *least two weeks:*
   1. **T**hought echo, insertion, withdrawal, broadcast
   2. Delusions of **C**ontrol, influence or passivity clearly referred to body or limb movements or specific thoughts, actions or sensations
   3. Hallucinatory **V**oices – running commentary, discussing the individual or other types of hallucinatory voices coming from some part of the body
   4. Persistent **D**elusions – culturally inappropriate and impossible, not just grandiose or persecutory
   5. Grossly **I**rrelevant/incoherent speech or frequent neologisms
   6. Intermittent or frequent appearance of some forms of **C**atatonic behaviour (e.g. waxy flexibility, posturing, negativism)

Irrelevant/incoherent speech
Control delusions
Affective disorders
Thought echo/insertion/withdrawal/broadcast
Voices
+
Catatonic behaviour
Delusions that are persistant
I C A TV & CD –*I see a TV and CD*

G3 G1 + G2 must be met in the same episode of the disorder, and concurrently for at least part of the episode
G4 Common exclusion criteria: organic mental disorder or psychoactive *substance misuse* disorder
N.B. Various types:

F25.0 Schizoaffective disorder, manic type

F25.1 Schizoaffective disorder, depressive type

F25.2 Schizoaffective disorder, mixed type

F25.8 Other schizoaffective disorders

F25.9 Schizoaffective disorder, unspecified

Note: *Timeline for psychotic disorders:*
Schizoaffective disorder (two weeks)
Acute psychotic disorder (<1 month)
Schizophrenia (one month)
Persistent delusional disorder (three months)

F28 Other non-organic psychotic disorders

F29 Unspecified non-organic psychosis

Summary

F20 General criteria for schizophrenia
CDs and **TVs** create a **NICHE**

F20.0 Paranoid schizophrenia
GAP

F20.1 Hebephrenic schizophrenia
ABCD

F20.2 Catatonic schizophrenia
SPAWNER

F20.4 Post-schizophrenic depression
GOAL

F20.5 Residual schizophrenia
REASON

F20.6 Simple schizophrenia
PENS

F21 Schizotypal disorder
RAPPORT

F22.0 Delusional disorder
DELUDE

F23 Acute and transient psychotic disorders
ACUTE

F23.0 Acute polymorphic disorder without symptoms of schizophrenia
RAPIDS

F23.1 Acute polymorphic disorder with symptoms of schizophrenia
A-DDS

F24 Induced delusional disorder
INDUCED

F25 Schizoaffective disorder
I C A CD & TV

Chapter 4
Mood disorders (F30–F39)

F30 Manic episode

All the subdivisions of this category must be used for a single episode. Hypomanic/manic episodes in those who have had 1/more previous affective episodes (depressive, hypomanic, manic or mixed) are coded as F31.- (bipolar affective disorder)

F30.0 Hypomania

A. Mood abnormally elevated/irritable for at _least four days_
B. 3/- of the following:
    i. Increased activity/restlessness/hyperactivity
    ii. Increased talkativeness/speech
    iii. Concentration/distractibility/'flipping' from idea to idea
    iv. Sleep reduced/insomnia
    v. Libido increased
    vi. Mild overspending
    vii. Increased sociability/overfamiliarity
C. The episode does not meet criteria for mania, anorexia nervosa, bipolar affective disorder (BAD), depressive episode, cyclothymia
D. Exclusion criteria – psychoactive substance use or organic mental disorder

Flipping from subject to subject/distractible
Overspending
Overfamiliar
Libido increased
Insomnia
Speech increased
Hyperactivity

Mood elevated for at least four days
Exclude other diagnoses (*see above*)

FOOLISH ME

F30.1 Mania without psychotic symptoms

A. Mood elevated/expansive/irritable and abnormal for the individual. This mood change is prominent and sustained for <u>at least one week</u>

B. At least 3/- of the following:
   i.   Activity increased
   ii.   Talkativeness (pressure of speech)
   iii. Flight of ideas (thoughts racing)
   iv. Sociability (loss of social inhibitions)
   v.   Insomnia (reduced need for sleep)
   vi. Grandiosity
   vii. Distractibility/constant changes in plans
   viii. Reckless behaviour
   ix. Sexual energy/libido

C. No hallucinations/delusions are present

D. Exclusion – psychoactive use and organic mental disorder

Distractibility
Insomnia
Grandiose

Flight of ideas
Activity increased
Sociability
Talkative
Energy (sexual) increased
Recklessness

DIG FASTER

F30.2 Mania with psychotic symptoms

Mania (F30.1) and psychotic symptoms, which include delusions (frequently grandiose) and/or hallucinations (usually voices talking directly to the individual)

OR:

Excitement, motor activity and flight of ideas are so extreme that the individual is incomprehensible
Mood congruent psychotic symptoms or
Mood incongruent psychotic symptoms or
Manic stupor

Exclusions include: schizophrenia, schizoaffective disorder (manic type), psychoactive substance use or organic mental disorder

F30.8 Other manic episodes

Mania, not otherwise specified (NOS)

F30.9 Manic episode, unspecified

F31 Bipolar affective disorder (BAD)

Two or more episodes where the individual's mood and activity are disturbed, specifically with an elevation in mood and activity *or* lowering of mood and decreased energy and activity. Repeated episodes of hypomania or mania only are classified under F31.8. Each episode is marked by a switch of an episode of the opposite or mixed episode or by remission

F31.0 Bipolar affective disorder, current episode hypomanic
Current episode hypomania, but the individual has had at least one other affective episode in the past (hypomanic, manic, depressive or mixed affective episode)

F31.1 Bipolar affective disorder, current episode manic without psychotic symptoms
Current episode manic, without psychotic symptoms and has had at least one affective episode in the past (hypomanic, manic, depressive or mixed affective episode)

F31.2 Bipolar affective disorder, current episode manic with psychotic symptoms
Psychotic symptoms can be either mood congruent or mood incongruent

F31.3 Bipolar affective disorder, current episode mild or moderate depression
With or without somatic syndrome

F31.4 Bipolar affective disorder, current episode severe depression without psychotic symptoms

F31.5 Bipolar affective disorder, current episode severe depression with psychotic symptoms
Psychotic symptoms can be either mood congruent or mood incongruent

F31.6 Bipolar affective disorder, current episode mixed
The individual has had one affective episode in the past and is currently exhibiting either a mixed or rapid alternation (within a few hours) of manic and depressive symptoms. Both manic and depressive symptoms should be prominent for most of the time during a period of at least two weeks

F31.7 Bipolar affective disorder currently in remission

F31.8 Other bipolar affective disorder
Includes bipolar II disorder and recurrent manic episodes

F31.9 Bipolar affective disorder unspecified

F32 Depressive episode

G1 The depressive episode lasts two weeks or longer
G2 There are no manic or hypomanic episodes previously
G3 Exclusion criteria: psychoactive and organic mental disorder

Somatic/biological syndrome includes four or more of the following:

Commences in the morning (depression worse in the morning)
Reduced emotional reactions/reactivity reduced
Appetite loss + interest in **A**ctivities lost
Weight loss (5% or more of bodyweight in the past month)
Libido loss
Early morning waking (two hours/more before usual time)
Retardation/agitation in psychomotor activity

CRA₂WLER

F32.0 Mild depressive episode
A. The general criteria for depressive disorder F32 met
B. At least two of (**LUE** *or* **ULE**):
    i.   Depressed mood for 2 weeks (**L**ow mood)
    ii.   Loss of interest/**U**ninterested in activities
    iii. **E**nergy decreased
C. Additional symptom(s) added to give a total of at <u>least four</u>:
    i.   **S**leep disturbance
    ii.   **A**ppetite change
    iii.   **G**uilt
    iv.   **E**steem reduced
    v.   **C**oncentration reduced
    vi.   **A**nd
    vii. **P**sychomotor activity change
    viii. **S**elf-harm/suicidal behaviour or thoughts

+/- Somatic syndrome (**CRA₂WLER**, fifth character used)

SAGE CaPSULE

'Sage capsules were previously used for treating depression'

F32.1 Moderate depressive episode
A. F32 general criteria must be met
B. At least two of **LUE**
C. Additional symptoms from F32.0 criterion C (**SAGE CaPS**) to give a total of at <u>least six</u>

+/- Somatic syndrome (**CRA₂WLER**, fifth character used)

F32.2 Severe depressive episode without psychotic symptoms
A. F32 general criteria must be met
B. All three of **LUE** met
C. Additional symptoms from F32.0 criterion C to give a total of at least eight
D. No hallucinations/delusions or depressive stupor

Somatic symptoms frequently present

F32.3 Severe depressive episode with psychotic symptoms
A. F32 general criteria must be met
B. Criteria for severe depressive episode without psychotic symptoms (F32.2) met apart from criterion D
C. Criterion for schizophrenia or schizoaffective depressive type not met
D. Either:
    i.   Hallucinations or delusions other than those typically seen in schizophrenia are present – commonly depressive, guilty, hypochondriachal, nihilistic, self-referential or persecutory in content
    ii.   Depressive stupor

A fifth character is used to identify whether psychotic symptoms are mood congruent or incongruent

F32.8 Other depressive episode
Including atypical and masked depression

F32.9 Depressive episode unspecified
Depression NOS
Depressive disorder NOS

F33 Recurrent depressive disorder

There is a history of repeated episodes of depression
There is a need to specify past severity

G1 At least **O**ne previous F32 episode mild/moderate/severe lasting at least two weeks
G2 At **N**o time – episode hypomania/manic
G3 **E**xclusion – psychoactive substance misuse or organic mental disorder

One (at least) previous depressive episode lasting at least two weeks
Never – manic/hypomanic
Exclusions

ONE

F33.0 Recurrent depressive disorder, current episode mild
A. General criteria for F33 met
B. Meets the criteria for mild depressive episode

+/- Somatic syndrome (**CRA$_2$WLER**, fifth character used)

Similar patterns for the following:

F33.1 Recurrent depressive disorder, current episode moderate
+/- Somatic syndrome

F33.2 Recurrent depressive disorder, current episode severe without psychotic symptoms

F33.3 Recurrent depressive disorder, current episode severe with psychotic symptoms
Psychotic symptoms can be either mood congruent or mood incongruent

F33.4 Recurrent depressive disorder, currently in remission
Recurrent depressive episodes (F33.0–33.3) in the past
Currently 'depression free' for *several months*

F33.8 Other recurrent depressive disorder

F33.9 Recurrent depressive disorder unspecified

F34 Persistent mood (affective) disorders

Does not meet criteria for depressive/hypomanic/manic episode
Can last for many years
Depressive and/or manic episodes can be superimposed on a persistent affective disorder

F34.0 Cyclothymia
A. At least two years of instability of mood involving periods of depression and hypomania
B. None of the manifestations in the two years meet the criteria for depressive/manic episode
C. When mood low, 3/- of the following:
Future worries
Insomnia
Interests reduced
No concentration
Esteem (self) low
Social withdrawal
Speech reduced
Energy reduced

FI₂NESSE

D. When mood elevated, 3/- of the following:
Interests increased
Gregarious
Overexaggerating
Talks/Witty banter increased
Energy increased
Esteem increased
Sleep - decreased need
Thinking sped up and more creative

I GO WEST

Two years + FINESSE + I GO WEST

'For finesse, I go West'

Can be classified as *early onset* or *late onset* depending on the age of first onset

F34.1 Dysthymia

A. At least two years of constant or recurring depressed mood
B. None or few episodes of depression (in the two-year period) that meet the criteria for recurrent mild depressive disorder (F33)
C. At least 3/- of the following:

Tearfulness
Energy + sexual activity reduced
Talkativeness reduced
Coping difficulties
Hopelessness + future
Interests reduced
No concentration
Esteem reduced
Social withdrawal
Sleep reduced

'**TETCHINESS** *can disguise dysthymia in clinical practice*'

Can be classified as *early onset* or *late onset* depending on the age of first onset

F34.8 Other persistent (affective) mood disorder
This is a residual disorder for those disorders not meeting criteria

F34.9 Persistent mood (affective) disorder unspecified

F38 Other mood (affective) disorders

F38.0 Other single mood [affective] disorders
F38.00 Mixed affective episode
A. **R**apid alternation of affective symptoms (within hours)
B. **B**oth manic and depressive symptoms are prominent (**A**ll affective disorders) most of the time for at least two weeks
C. **N**o previous history of hypomanic, depressive or mixed episodes

Rapid alternation of symptoms
All affective disorders present
No past history of hypomania, depressive or mixed episodes

RAN

F38.1 Other recurrent mood [affective] disorders

F38.10 Recurrent brief depressive disorder
A. Meets the criteria for mild/moderate/severe depressive episode
B. Occurs once a month over the past year
C. Each episode lasts <2 weeks (usually 2–3 days)
D. Unrelated to any physiological changes, e.g. a menstrual cycle

Short episodes (<2 weeks)
Unrelated to physiological changes
Meets criteria for a depressive episode
Once a month; every year

SUMO

F38.8 Other specified mood disorder

F39 Unspecified mood (affective) disorder

Affective psychosis, NOS

Summary

F30.0 Hypomania
FOOLISH ME

F30.1 Mania without psychotic symptoms
DIG FASTER

F32 Depressive episode
CRA$_2$WLER

F32.0 Mild depressive episode
SAGE CaPSULE

F33 Recurrent depressive disorder
ONE

F34.0 Cyclothymia
Two years + FINESSE + I GO WEST

F34.1 Dysthymia
TETCHINESS

F38.00 Mixed affective disorders
RAN

F38.1 Recurrent brief depressive disorder
SUMO

Chapter 5

Neurotic, stress-related and somatoform disorders (F40–F48)

Whilst not in the diagnostic classification, Marks (1970) described abnormal fears as:
1. *Class one* – phobias of external stimuli (agoraphobia, social phobia, animal and other specific phobias)
2. *Class two* – phobias of internal stimuli (illness and obsessive phobias)

F40 Phobic anxiety disorders

A group of disorders in which anxiety is created in certain well-defined situations that are not necessarily dangerous. Contemplating the phobic situation generates anticipatory anxiety. The individual's focus may be on symptoms such as palpitations or dry mouth, etc.

F40.0 Agoraphobia
A group of disorders involving a fear of leaving home, entering shops, crowds and public places or travelling alone in trains, buses or planes. Frequently associated with panic disorder

A. Fear/avoidance of at least two of the following:
   i.   Crowds
   ii. Travelling alone
   iii. Public places
   iv. Travelling away from home

Travelling – away from home or alone
Crowds
Public places

TCP

B. 2/- of the following:
ABCO (Autonomic, Brain, Chest & Others)
<u>Autonomic (think **pulse**)</u>
Palpitations
Unsteady hands/tremor
Lack of saliva
Sweat, **E**xcess

PULSE

<u>Brain related</u>
Balance affected/dizzy
Reality questioned (derealisation (objects unreal) and depersonalisation (feeling unreal))
And
Impending doom/death
No longer in control

BRAIN

<u>Chest/abdomen</u>
Choking feeling
HEart pain
Stomach churning + nausea
Tachypnoea (breathing difficulty)

CHEST

Don't forget the Others!
Hot flushes/cold chills
Numbness/tingling sensations

C. Emotional distress – caused by Avoidance or by anxiety symptoms
D. Anxieties predominate in the feared *situations* or the *contemplation* of the feared situations
E. Exclude other mental disorders

Note:
Feared Situations: **TCP**
Symptoms: **ABCO**
General: Avoidance + Anxiety + Exclusions
Can exist with or without <u>panic disorder</u>

F40.1 Social phobias

A. Either:
   i. Fear of being the focus of attention or fear of behaving in a way that will be humiliating; or
   ii. Avoidance of being the centre of attention or of situations where there will be fear of behaving in an embarrassing way
B. Criterion B of F40.0 together with at least 1/- of the following:
   i. Blushing/shaking
   ii. Fear of vomiting
   iii. Urgency/fear of micturition or defaecation
C. Emotional distress caused by avoidance or anxiety symptoms
D. An understanding that symptoms or avoidance are unreasonable
E. Anxieties predominate in the feared *situations* or the *contemplation* of the feared situations
F. Exclusions – organic mental disorder, schizophrenia and related disorders, obsessive-compulsive disorders.

Fear of object/situation
Emotional distress
Avoidance of object/situation
Restricted anxiety to feared situations or contemplation of the situation
Symptoms: ABCO (i.e. criterion B of F40.0) plus additional symptoms

FEARS

F40.2 Specific phobias

A. Either:
   i. Marked <u>fear</u> of a specific object/situation not described in F40.0–40.1, or
   ii. Marked <u>avoidance</u> of a specific object/situation not described in F40.0–40.1
B. Symptoms of anxiety in the feared situations described in criterion B of F40.0 (ABCO)
C. Emotional distress is caused by the symptoms or the avoidance
D. Symptoms restricted to the feared situations or contemplation of the feared situation

Specific phobias can be subdivided into various sections: Animals, Nature, Blood, Injections, Situational or others

F40.8 Other phobic anxiety disorders

F40.9 Phobic anxiety disorder, unspecified
Phobia NOS or phobic state NOS

F41 Other anxiety disorders

F41.0 Panic disorder
Recurrent attacks of severe anxiety unrestricted to any situation or set of circumstances that are *unpredictable*
It can be a *secondary* feature of an affective disorder
Excludes Agoraphobia with panic disorder (F40.0)

A. Recurrent panic attacks
B. Panic attack characterised by:
    i.   Discrete episodes
    ii. Abrupt onset
    iii. Peak within a few minutes and last a few minutes
    iv. At least four symptoms of **ABCO** (*see p. 74*)
C. Exclusions, e.g. physical health problem or other mental disorder

Secondary feature of an affective disorder occasionally
Time – several minutes
Recurrent
Episodic + Exclusions
Abrupt onset
Multiple symptoms

STREAM
+
ABCO (*see above*)

F41.1 Generalised anxiety disorder (GAD)
A. At least six months of tension, worry and feeling of apprehension about everyday events and problems
B. 4/- of symptoms:
    i.   **ABC** (*see p. 74*)
    ii. General:
    Hot flushes/chills
    Numbness/tingling sensations
    Muscle tension/pains
    Restlessness
    Feeling on edge
    Difficulty in swallowing

Restlessness
Edgy
Swallowing difficulties
Temperature fluctuations – hot flushes/chills
Sensation changes – tension/pains + numbness/tingling

RESTS
   iii.   Others:
Poor **SL**eep
Irritability
Poor **C**oncentration
Exaggerated startle response

SLICE

C. Does not meet the criteria for panic disorder, phobic anxiety disorders, obsessive-compulsive disorder or hypochondriachal disorder
D. Exclude other disorders – physical disorder, e.g. hyperthyroidism, psychoactive substance misuse disorder or organic mental disorder

Generalised worries
Edginess
No control over anxieties
Excess sweat
Restlessness
Attention/concentration deficits
Lack of saliva
Irritability
Sleep poor
Energy decreased
Deep tension in muscles

GENERALISED

A useful aid to remember some of the significant symptoms of GAD

F41.2 Mixed anxiety and depressive disorder
Symptoms of depression and anxiety both present
Neither one is predominant or meets criteria for an individual diagnosis

F41.3 Other mixed anxiety disorders
Includes symptoms of an anxiety disorder with features of F42–F48, but does not meet the criteria for an individual diagnosis

F41.8 Other specified anxiety disorders

F41.9 Anxiety disorder, unspecified
Anxiety disorder, NOS

F42 Obsessive-compulsive disorder

A. Obsessions or compulsions (or both) for most days for two weeks or more
B. Obsessions (thoughts/ideas/images) and compulsions (acts) present as:
   i.   Originating in the mind of the individual
   ii.   Repetitive and unpleasant
   iii.   Patient tries to resist them
   iv.   The experience of carrying out the act or having the thought is Unpleasant
C. The obsession/compulsion causes distress/interferes with the individual's functioning, usually by being time consuming
D. Exclusions, e.g. schizophrenia or affective disorder

Repetitive
Experience is unpleasant
Patient tries to resist
Originates in mind
Rule out others (*see above*)
Two weeks' duration
Slowness

REPORTS

F42.0 Predominantly obsessional thoughts or ruminations
Ideas/images/impulses that are usually distressing for the individual

F42.1 Predominantly compulsive acts
Usually to do with cleaning, repeated checking, tidiness or orderliness. The purpose of the ritual is to avert any potential danger

F42.2 Mixed obsessional thoughts and acts

F42.8 Other obsessive-compulsive disorders

F42.9 Obsessive-compulsive disorder, unspecified

F43 Reactions to severe stress and adjustment disorders

F43.0 Acute stress reaction

A. The individual is exposed to an exceptional stressor (physical or mental)
B. Onset of symptoms is usually within an hour following exposure to the stressor
C. Acute stress reaction graded – mild/moderate/severe
D. Symptoms reduce after 8 (if a transient stressor) – 48 hours (if stressor continues)
E. Other diagnoses excluded

Stress exposure
TRansient by nature (reduce after 8–48 hours)
Exclude other disorders
Symptoms appear after an hour
Severity graded – mild/moderate/severe

STRESS

F43.1 Post-traumatic stress disorder

A. **E**xposure to a stressful event/situation that is exceptionally threatening/catastrophic in nature
B. **R**eliving of the stressor – flashbacks, vivid memories or dreams
C. **A**voidance of situations associated with the stressor
D. **H**yperarousal:
   i. Inability to recall aspects the stressful event; and/or
   ii. Persisting symptoms of psychological arousal, i.e. insomnia/irritability/hypervigilance/exaggerated startle/poor concentration
E. The criteria met within six months of the stressful event (**B**efore six months after exposure) – this can be longer but this needs to be specified

Reliving of the stressor
Exposure to a stressful event
Hyperaroused
Avoidance
Before six months – criteria met

REHAB

F43.2 Adjustment disorders

A. Symptoms occur within one month of the stressor
B. Symptoms manifest themselves as an affective disorder (F30–F39) (other than any psychotic manifestation), for example:
   i.   Brief depressive reaction
   ii.   Prolonged depressive reaction
   iii. Mixed anxiety and depressive reaction (amongst other subtypes)
C. Except in a prolonged depressive reaction, symptoms *do not exceed six months*

Six months' maximum duration
Affective disorder manifestation
Duration within one month of the stressor

SAD

F43.8 Other reactions to severe stress

F43.9 Reaction to severe stress, unspecified

F44 Dissociative (conversion) disorders

Frequently, there is partial or complete *loss of the normal integration* between memories of the past, awareness of identity and immediate sensations, and control of bodily movements
Loss (partial or complete) of the normal integration between:

Past **R**ecall
Identity awareness
Sensation awareness
Movements

PRISM

G1 No evidence of a physical disorder explaining the symptoms
G2 There is a convincing association between the onset of symptoms and stressful events

F44.0 Dissociative amnesia
A. General criteria for F44 are met
B. Amnesia (partial/complete) for **R**ecent events or problems that were or are still traumatic or stressful
C. **A**mnesia much more **E**xtensive than that explained by forgetfulness/simulation

If the amnesia is complete and generalised, there is a need to consider dissociative fugue. This is not attributable to another disorder such as a psychoactive-related disorder

Extensive **A**mnesia
Recent events especially

EAR

F44.1 Dissociative fugue
A. General criteria for F44 met
B. The person takes an unexpected **J**ourney away from home or work, during which self-care is maintained
C. **A**mnesia (partial/complete) for *the journey*, which **M**eets criteria C of dissociative amnesia (F44.0)

Journey away from home
Amnesia – partial/complete
Meets criteria C of F44.0

JAM

'Getting into a jam'

F44.2 Dissociative stupor
A. General criteria for F44 met
B. Profound diminution/absence of voluntary movements, speech and normal responsiveness to light, noise and touch
C. Normal muscle tone, posture and breathing are maintained

Speech reduced
Tone normal
Unable to move
Posture normal
Otherwise normal responsiveness to light, etc.
Respiration maintained

STUPOR

F44.3 Trance and possession disorders
A. General criteria for F44 met
B. Either:
   i. Trance disorder – temporary alteration of the state of consciousness; or
   ii. Possession disorder – convinced he/she has been taken over by a spirit/someone else/other power
C. Both criteria are difficult to manage and occur outside cultural norms
D. Exclusion – schizophrenia or affective disorders with hallucinations or delusions

Trance + **P**ossession disorders
Away from cultural norms and other diagnoses

TAP

F44.4 Dissociative motor disorders
A. General criteria for F44 met
B. Either:
   i. Complete/partial loss of the ability to perform movements normally under voluntary control; or
   ii. Some other features relating to inco-ordination/ataxia or inability to stand unaided

F44.5 Dissociative convulsions
Differentiated from epilepsy from the above
There may be other methods that suggest a non-epileptic rationale for the episodes

A. General criteria for F44 met
B. Sudden and spasmodic movements resembling epileptic seizures but no loss of consciousness
C. Not accompanied by tongue biting, serious bruising, laceration or injury from falling or urinary incontinence

F44.6 Dissociative anaesthesia and sensory loss
A. General criteria for F44 met
B. Either:
    i. Partial/complete loss of normal cutaneous sensations over usually part/all of body; or
    ii. Partial/complete loss of vision, hearing or smell

F44.7 Mixed dissociative (conversion) disorders

F44. 8 Other dissociative (conversion) disorders

F44.80 Ganser's syndrome
Think *Ganser –sounds like 'Answer'* (approximate answers)

F44.81 Multiple personality disorder
The key feature is the apparent presence of two or more distinct personalities within an individual, with only one of them being evident at a time. Change between one personality to another is often triggered by a stressful experience. This is a rare, controversial condition, with most cases occurring in North America

A. Two or more distinct personality disorders existing in the same person with only one evident at a time
B. Each personality has its own memories/behaviour patterns with episodic full control of the individual
C. Inability to recall personal information – too extensive to be described as normal forgetfulness
D. Exclusions – organic or psychoactive-related disorder

Multiple personalities, two or more

USA – more frequently seen in North America (not a diagnostic feature)

Lack of alternative explanation for behaviour

Total control of an individual episodically

Inability to recall personal information

MULTI

F44.9 Dissociative (conversion) disorder unspecified

F45 Somatoform disorder

F45.0 Somatisation disorder
The main feature includes repeated complaints of a physical nature together with a persistent request for medical investigations despite persistent negative findings

A. A two-year history of persisting complaints of multiple and variable physical symptoms unexplained by any detectable physical disorders
B. Preoccupation with symptoms leads to distress, leading the individual to repeatedly seek out medical advice/investigations or self-medicate with various remedies
C. Persistent refusal to accept medical reassurance that there is no underlying physical cause
D. A number of physical health symptoms:
    i.   Gastrointestinal
    ii. Cardiovascular
    iii. Genitourinary
    iv. Skin and pain syndromes/Cutaneous

GC GC
E. Exclusion criteria – F20–F29, F30–F39, F41

Symptom groups (**GC GC**)
Unexplained symptoms
Refusal to accept reassurance
Preoccupation with symptoms
Symptoms Into Second year
Exclusions

SURPrISE

Somatisation disorder frequently leaves physicians 'surprised'

F45.1 Undifferentiated somatoform disorder
Somatoform complaints that are *multiple, varying and persistent*
The complete criteria for somatisation disorder not met
Duration for at least six months

F45.2 Hypochondriachal disorder
A. Either:
  i. Persistent preoccupation (six months' duration) with 1–2 serious physical diseases; or
  ii. Persistent preoccupation with a presumed deformity (body dysmorphic disorder)
B. Preoccupation with symptoms leads to distress, leading the individual to repeatedly seek out medical advice/investigations or self-medicate with various remedies
C. Refusal to accept medical advice
D. Exclude others
N.B. Depression + anxiety frequently present

Preoccupation with a physical disorder or deformity
Unipolar depression or other affective or anxiety disorders frequently present
Refusal to accept medical advice
Seeks medical advice repeatedly
Exclude other psychiatric causes

PURSE

An individual uses their 'purse' to pay for repeated investigations/medical opinions

F45.3 Somatoform autonomic dysfunction (SAD)
This is a disorder relating to symptoms of autonomic arousal that are attributed to a physical disorder or organ, largely or completely under autonomic control (gastrointestinal, genitourinary, cardiovascular, respiratory and urogenital systems)
Includes a variety of (objective) autonomic arousal symptoms including palpitations, sweating, dry mouth, epigastric discomfort
Subjective complaints often of a changing nature, which are referred by the patient to a specific organ or system

Subjective complaints of a changing nature
Autonomic arousal
Diverse range of symptoms

SAD

F45.4 Persistent somatoform pain disorder

There are complaints of persistent and severe pain for at least six months. This is not explained by evidence of a physical disorder or physiological process

Exclusion criteria – Schizophrenia and related disorders (F20–F29), Affective disorders (F30–F39), Somatisation disorder (F45.0), Undifferentiated somatoform disorder (F45.1) or Hypochondraical disorder (F45.2)

F45.8 Other somatoform disorders

Any other disorders of sensation/function/behaviour not due to physical disorders and not mediated through the autonomic nervous system

The symptoms are often closely associated in time with stressful events or problems

The outcome often results in increased attention for the patient

F45.9 Somatoform disorder, unspecified

Includes psychosomatic disorder NOS

F48 Other neurotic disorders

F48.0 Neurasthenia

Persistent and distressing complaints of exhaustion after minor mental effort; or

Persistent and distressing complaints of feelings of fatigue and weakness after minor physical effort

Rest or relaxation does not help the above

Including a variety of unpleasant symptoms (at least one, *excluding irritability):

Sleep disturbance
Tension headaches
Aches and pains (muscular)
Irritability* (this is usually present)
Relaxation problems
Staggering/dizziness

STAIRS

'Even stairs are difficult in neurasthenia'

Exclude – Organic emotionally labile disorder (F06.6), Postencephalitic syndrome (F07.1), Postconcussional syndrome (F07.2), Affective disorders (F30–F39), Panic disorder (F41.0) or Generalised anxiety disorder (F41.1)

Lasts at least six months

F48.1 Depersonalisation-derealisation syndrome

A. Either:
    i.   Depersonalisation – feelings of being distant or unreal; or
    ii. Derealisation – feelings that the world is unreal
B. Insight retention – the patient realises that he/she is not being imposed upon by outside forces

Must be differentiated from other mental disorders, such as organic or psychotic disorders

F48.8 Other specified neurotic disorders

Includes: Dhat, Koro and Latah. These are not viewed as delusional because of their cultural influence

F48.9 Neurotic disorder, unspecified

Summary

F40.0 Agoraphobia
Feared situations: **TCP**
Symptoms: **ABCO**

F40.1 Social phobias
FEARS

F41.0 Panic disorder
STREAM (+ ABC & O)

F41.1 Generalised anxiety disorder (GAD)
GENERALISED

F43.0 Acute stress reaction
STRESS

F43.1 Post-traumatic stress disorder
REHAB

F43.2 Adjustment disorders
SAD

F44.0 Dissociative amnesia
EAR

F44.1 Dissociative fugue
JAM

F44.2 Dissociative stupor
STUPOR

F44.3 Trance and possession disorders
TAP

F44.81 Multiple personality disorder
MULTI

F45.0 Somatisation disorder
SURPriSE

F45.2 Hypochondriachal disorder
PURSE

F48.0 Neurasthenia
STAIRS

Reference

Marks IM. The classification of phobic disorders. *Br J Psychiatry.* 1970; **116**: 377–86.

Chapter 6

Behavioural syndromes associated with physiological disturbances and physical factors (F50–F59)

F50 Eating disorders

F50.0 Anorexia nervosa (AN)
Weight loss – 15% below normal/expected weight
Exclude bulimia nervosa or others
Intrusive dread related to fatness
*Gym work and other methods employed to lose weight (*suggestive not diagnostic*)
Hypothalamic-pituitary-gonadal axis alteration – amenorrhoea/loss of sexual interest
Turns down/avoids (perceived) fatty foods

WEIGHT

Supportive (but not diagnostic) factors include:

Self-induced vomiting
Purging
Appetite suppressant use
Diuretic or
Excessive exercise

SPADE

F50.1 Atypical anorexia nervosa
Fulfil some but not all features of AN

F50.2 Bulimia nervosa (BN)
Binge eating – at least twice a week over three months
Urge/compulsion to eat
Let me starve – alternating periods of starvation
Intrusive dread of fatness
Many methods of counteracting fatness including:
Induced vomiting
Appetite suppression

BULIMIA

F50.3 Atypical bulimia nervosa
Fulfil some but not all features of BN, so that the clinical picture does not justify a diagnosis of BN

F50.4 Overeating associated with other psychological disturbances
Overeating that is secondary to stressful events, e.g. bereavement

F50.5 Vomiting associated with other psychological disturbances
Vomiting associated with dissociative disorders and hypochondriachal disorder

F50.8 Other eating disorders
For example, pica in adults and psychogenic loss of appetite

F50.9 Eating disorder unspecified
Eating disorder, NOS

F51 Non-organic sleep disorders

Essentially, a disturbance of sleep felt to be a condition in itself and not secondary to any other causes

F51.0 Non-organic insomnia
Falling asleep/maintaining/non-refreshing sleep problem
All other disorders excluded, i.e. medical, psychoactive or medication
Interference with daily living
Three times a week for at least a month
however, children – not coded here

FAITh

F51.1 Non-organic hypersomnia
Sleepiness during daytime/sleep attacks/sleep disturbance
Every day for at least one month
All other disorders excluded – medical, psychoactive or medication induced
No other symptoms of narcolepsy or evidence of sleep apnoea

SEAN ... *the sleepy sheep(!)*

F51.2 Non-organic disorder of the sleep-wake cycle
Interference with life
Disorder of sleep-wake cycle
Every day for at least one month
All other disorders excluded – medical, psychoactive or medication induced

IDEA

F51.3 Sleep walking/somnambulism
Walking for several minutes – half an hour
All others disorders excluded – medical, psychoactive or medication induced
Limited communication following the episode – awakened with considerable difficulty
Knowledge limited about the episode (amnesia)
Short period of confusion after episode

WALKS

F51.4 Sleep terrors

All other disorders excluded – medical, psychoactive or medication induced

First third of sleep

Recall limited for event + response to comfort is poor

Anxiety and autonomic hyperactivity – 2+ episodes

Individual lacks response followed by disorientation

Duration is less than 10 minutes

AFRAID

F51.5 Nightmares

Marked anxiety on awakening in response from dreams but then alert/orientated

All other disorders excluded – medical, psychoactive or medication induced

Recall is present

Experience is distressing

Second half of sleep is usually when nightmares occur

MARES

F51.8 Other non-organic sleep disorders

F51.9 Non-organic sleep disorder, unspecified

For example, emotional sleep disorder

F52 Sexual dysfunction, not caused by organic disorder or disease

General criteria:
Frequently occurs in the individual but can be absent on some occasions
Unable to participate in a sexual relationship
Six months at least
Exclusion of other disorders (mental and physical)

FUSE

F52.0 Lack or loss of sexual desire
Loss of sexual desire is the primary problem and is not secondary to any other disorder, for example erectile dysfunction. Meets the criteria for F52

Lack of **I**nterest in initiating sexual activity
Lack/loss of sexual **D**esire

ID

F52.1 Sexual aversion and lack of sexual enjoyment
Idea of sexual activity causes anxiety – sexual aversion (F52.10)
If sexual responses occur with no difficulty but there is *no resulting pleasure*, this is lack of sexual enjoyment (F52.11)

F52.2 Failure of genital response
The primary problem in men is erectile dysfunction
The primary problem for women is lubrication failure: **F**ema**L**e

F52.3 Orgasmic dysfunction
Orgasm either:
1. Does not occur; or
2. Is very delayed
N.B. There are further subtypes based on contextual factors

F52.4 Premature ejaculation
This is the failure to control ejaculation as part of normal sexual activity

F52.5 Non-organic vaginismus
Spasm of the pelvic floor muscles causing closure of the vaginal opening due to a psychogenic cause

F52.6 Non-organic dyspareunia
This is used for when there is pain during sexual intercourse occurring in men and women. Used when there is no primary non-organic sexual dysfunction, which includes vaginismus/vaginal dryness

F52.7 Excessive sexual drive
Includes nymphomania and satyriasis

F52.8 Other sexual dysfunction not caused by organic disorder

F52.9 Unspecified sexual dysfunction not caused by organic disorder or disease

F53 Mental and behavioural disorders associated with the puerperium, not elsewhere classified

This is a category for disorders occurring in the puerperium (occurring within six weeks of the delivery). The disorders listed in this section do not meet any other disorders listed elsewhere

F53.0 Mild mental and behavioural disorders associated with the puerperium, not elsewhere classified
Depression postnatal NOS or postpartum NOS

F53.1 Severe mental and behavioural disorders associated with the puerperium, not elsewhere classified
Puerperal psychosis NOS

F53.8 Other mental and behavioural disorders, not otherwhere classified

F53.9 Puerperal mental disorder, unspecified

F54 Psychological and behavioural factors associated with disorders or diseases classified elsewhere

This is a category used for psychological factors affecting physical disorders, e.g. asthma, gastric ulcer or ulcerative colitis and others. The associated mental disorder should be mild, limiting and must not fulfil criteria for another mental and behavioural disorder

Example: for asthma, F54 and J45 (the ICD-10 code for asthma)

F55 Abuse of non-dependence-producing substances

This includes the use of a variety of different medications and whilst there is a <u>strong desire</u> to take the medications, there is <u>no evidence of dependence</u>. The most common substances include antidepressants, diuretics, laxatives and analgesics

F55.0 Antidepressants

F55.1 Analgesics

F55.3 Antacids

F55.4 Vitamins

F55.5 Steroids or hormones

F55.6 Specific herbal or folk remedies

F55.8 Other substances that do not produce dependence

F55.9 Unspecified behavioural syndromes associated with physiological disturbances and physical factors
Psychogenic-physiological dysfunction, NOS

Summary

F50.0 Anorexia nervosa (AN)
WEIGHT

F50.2 Bulimia nervosa (BN)
BULIMIA

F51.0 Non-organic insomnia
FAITh

F51.1 Non-organic hypersomnia
SEAN ... the sleepy sheep(!)

F51.2 Non-organic disorder of the sleep-wake cycle
IDEA

F51.3 Sleep walking/somnambulism
WALKS

F51.4 Sleep terrors
AFRAID

F51.5 Nightmares
MARES

F52 Sexual dysfunction, not caused by organic disorder or disease
FUSE

F52.0 Lack or loss of sexual desire
ID

F52.2 Failure of genital response
The primary problem in m<u>e</u>n is <u>e</u>rectile dysfunction
The primary problem for women is lubrication failure: <u>F</u>ema<u>L</u>e

Chapter 7

Disorders of adult personality and behaviour (F60–F69)

F60 Specific personality disorders (PD)

General personality disorder criteria (G1–G6) *must* be fulfilled before a specific personality disorder is diagnosed

G1
One or more difficulties in the following areas:

Control over impulses/gratification
Relating to others
Affectivity
Cognition/knowledge

CRACk

G2
Pervasive **B**ehaviour that is maladaptive over a range of different situations

G3
Personal **D**istress/adverse impact on social environment

G4
Onset in late childhood/**A**dolescence

G5
Not explained by any **O**ther mental disorder

G6
Not as a result of **O**rganic brain injury/disease

Behaviour
Adolescent onset
Distress

Control over impulses
Relating to others
Organic/other disorders not responsible
Affectivity
Cognition/**k**nowledge

BAD CROACk (G1–G6)

Specific personality disorder types
Note that in each disorder, the general criteria for personality disorder F60 (G1–G6) should be fulfilled

F60.0 Paranoid personality disorder
Four of the following:

Spouse fidelity questioned
Unforgotten grudges – refuses to ignore/forgive insults
Suspiciousness
Personal rights paramount
Excessive self-importance and self-referential attitude
Conspiratorial explanations of events
Threats perceived in everyday events
Sensitivity to setbacks or criticism

SUSPECTS

F60.1 Schizoid personality disorder
Four of the following:

Pleasure from activities limited
Emotional coldness
Consistent choice for solitary activities
Uninterested in having sexual relations
Limited capacity to express feelings
Insensitivity to social norms
Appears indifferent to praise/criticism
References to fantasy and introspection
Social network/friendships limited

PECULIARS

F60.2 Dissocial personality disorder
Three of the following:

Callous unconcern for others
Regard for social norms is minimal
Incapacity for guilt
Maintenance of relationships is poor
Everyone else to blame
Self-control – poor tolerance of frustration

CRIMES

F60.3 Emotionally unstable personality disorder

F60.30 Impulsive type

Three of the following:

Suddenly act (unexpectedly)
Capricious mood
Outbursts of anger/violence
Liable to quarrel
Difficulty maintaining course of action when there is no reward

SCOLD

F60.31 Borderline type

Three of the following:

Perceived self-image problems
Liability to be involved in intense and unstable relationships
Emptiness feelings
Abandonment
Self-harm – either thoughts or acts

PLEAS

F60.4 Histrionic personality disorder

Four of the following:

Provocative behaviour/seductiveness
Risqué (physical) appearance
Affectivity shallow and labile
Influenced easily
Self-dramatisation
Excitement is sought by being the centre of attention

PRAISE

F60.5 Anankastic personality disorder

Four of the following:

Social conventions and rules strictly adhered to
Loses point of activities due to preoccupation with detail, roles and schedules
Overly perfectionist attitude interferes with tasks
Worries, doubts and caution

Friendships limited due to preoccupation with work/productivity
Inflexible attitude
Reluctant to delegate
Meticulousness in tasks

SLOW FIRM

F60.6 Anxious (avoidant) personality disorder
Four of the following:

Certainty of being liked before being involved with others
Rejection or criticism is the main preoccupation
Interpersonal relationships avoided due to perceived shame
Keeps avoiding occupational and social activities (involving significant interpersonal contact)
Embarrassment/apprehension/tension prevents new activities
'You're unappealing' – self-belief

CRIKEY

F60.7 Dependent personality disorder
Four of the following:

Decision-making difficulty without advice from others
Excessive lengths to obtain support from others with subordination of own needs
Preoccupation about abandonment
Exaggerated fears of being unable to care for himself or herself
Needs others to assume responsibility for his or her life
Difficulty expressing disagreement with others

DEPEND

F60.8 Other specific personality disorder

F60.9 Personality disorder, unspecified

F61 Mixed and other personality disorder

Intended for personality disorders that are often troublesome but do not demonstrate the specific pattern of symptoms that characterise the disorders in F60

F61.0 Mixed personality disorders

F61.1 Troublesome personality changes

F62 Enduring personality changes not attributable to brain damage and disease

This group includes disorders of adult personality and behaviour that have developed in persons with no previous personality disorder, following exposure to a catastrophic or excessively prolonged stress, or a severe psychiatric illness

F62.0 Enduring personality change after catastrophic experience
Personality changes after exposure to a catastrophic or excessive prolonged stress, or following a severe psychiatric illness. Personality changes must have been present for two years following exposure to catastrophic stress. Post-traumatic stress disorder often precedes this diagnosis

F62.1 Enduring personality change after psychiatric illness
This group includes personality change, persisting for at least two years, attributable to the traumatic experience of suffering from a severe psychiatric illness

F62.8 Other enduring personality changes
Including chronic pain personality syndrome

F62.9 Enduring personality change unspecified

F63 Habit and impulse disorders

Includes certain disorders of behaviour not classified under other categories. They are characterised by repeated acts that have no clear rational motivation and harm the individual's own interests and those of others

F63.0 Pathological gambling

Consists of two or more episodes of gambling over a year. The episodes do not have profitable outcome but are continued despite personal distress and interference with daily living. There is an intense urge to gamble, which is difficult to control

2/+ episodes/year
Pre**O**ccupation
Urge that is intense
No profit
Distress

2 PoUND (think cash/£)

F63.1 Pathological fire-setting (pyromania)

Consists of two or more episodes with no apparent motive and intense urges to set fire to objects (urge for fire). There is a preoccupation with thoughts or images of the fire-setting or the circumstances surrounding the act

2/+ episodes/year
Pre**O**ccupation
Urge
For
Fire

2 PUFF (think 'puff' of smoke)

F63.2 Pathological stealing (kleptomania)

Consists of **two** or more thefts where the individual steals without any apparent motive or gain
Intense **U**rge to **S**teal (US)

2 US (thieves steal from 'us')

F63.3 Trichotillomania
Noticeable hair loss as a result of the impulses to pull hair

No other reason for the behaviour
Urge to pull out hairs
Lots of **L**oss

NULL (*left with little or 'null' hair*)

F63.8 Other habit and impulse disorder
Other kinds of persistently repeated maladaptive behaviour that are not secondary to another psychiatric syndrome

F64 Gender identity disorders

F64.0 Transsexualism
Note the 'sex' part, i.e. gender – where an individual wishes to live as a member of the opposite sex. The transsexual desire ought to be present for at *least two years* and should not originate from another mental disorder (for example, schizophrenia)

F64.1 Dual-role transvestism
Note the *'vest'* part (i.e. clothing). This is the wearing of clothes of the opposite sex to enjoy the brief membership of the opposite sex, with no desire for a permanent gender change or sexual excitement

F64.2 Gender identity disorder of childhood (GID)
Develops in early childhood (before puberty) and is characterised by a persistent and intense distress about the assigned gender together with a desire to be the other sex. The behaviours identified must be more than mere tomboyishness in girls or girlish behaviour in boys and should be present for at least six months

Gender causes
Intense
Distress

GID

F64.8 Other gender identity disorders

F64.9 Gender identity disorder, unspecified

F65 Disorders of sexual preference

General criteria:
Intense sexual urges involving objects/fantasies
Individual acts on urges or is distressed by them
Preference has been present for at least six months

O – objects
D – distress
D – duration at least six months

ODD

F65.0 Fetishism
Reliance on a non-living object as a stimulus for sexual arousal and gratification. Frequently limited to males only

F65.1 Fetishistic transvestism
<u>Fetish</u> + <u>Transvestism</u>
This is the wearing of clothes of the opposite sex to create sexual excitement and in order to create the appearance of a person from the opposite sex. Distinguished (from transvestism) by the presence of sexual arousal and the removal of clothing after orgasm is reached

F65.2 Exhibitionism
A recurrent or persistent tendency to expose genitals to strangers, usually of the opposite sex, or to people in public places. There is no intention to have sexual intercourse with the witness, but the act is frequently associated with sexual arousal and masturbation

F65.3 Voyeurism
A recurrent or persistent tendency to look at people engaging in sexual or intimate behaviour. This is carried out without the observed being aware and usually leads to sexual excitement, e.g. masturbation. There is no intention for sexual intercourse with the observed individuals

F65.4 Paedophilia
A persistent sexual preference for children, usually of prepubertal age. The individual must be at least 16 years old and at least five years older than the child or children

F65.5 Sadomasochism

A preference for sexual activity which involves pain, humiliation or bondage

If a provider = <u>sadism</u>

If a recipient = <u>masochism</u>

Frequently individuals obtain sexual excitement from *both* sadistic and masochistic activities

F65.6 Multiple disorders of sexual preference

More than one abnormal sexual preference occurs in one person

F65.8 Other disorders of sexual preference

Includes a variety of other patterns of sexual preference, e.g. frottism

F65.9 Disorder of sexual preference unspecified

F66 Psychological and behavioural disorders

This section is for descriptive purposes to illustrate variations of sexual development. Sexual orientation is not to be regarded as a disorder

F66.0 Sexual maturation disorder
The individual suffers from uncertainty about his or her:
1. Gender identity; or
2. Sexual orientation causing anxiety or depression

Most often seen in adolescents or those in stable relationships finding that their orientation is changing

F66.1 Egodystonic sexual orientation
The gender identity or sexual preference is not in doubt, but the individual wishes it were different because of associated psychological and behavioural disorders and may seek treatment to change it

F66.2 Sexual relationship disorder
The gender identity or sexual preference is responsible for the difficulties in the sexual relationship

F66.8 Other psychosexual development disorders

F66.9 Psychosexual development disorder, unspecified

F68 Other disorders of adult personality and behaviour

F68.0 Elaboration of physical symptoms for psychological reasons

Physical symptoms originally due to a confirmed physical disorder become prolonged in excess of what was expected. There is also evidence of a psychological causation for the excessive symptoms (includes compensation neurosis)

F68.1 Intentional production or feigning of symptoms or disabilities, ether physical or psychological (factitious disorder)

Feigning symptoms repeatedly for no obvious reasons and may even self-inflict wounds in order to produce symptoms

There is no evidence of external motivation (for example, financial compensation)

Distinguished from malingering as this (F68.1) is *not* goal related

If there is a mental or physical disorder that could explain the symptoms, this diagnosis is not made

F68.8 Other specified disorders of adult personality and behaviour

Includes: Character disorder, NOS, and Relationship disorder, NOS

F69 Unspecified disorder of adult personality and behaviour

Only used as a last resort, if the presence of a disorder of adult personality and behaviour can be assumed but information to confirm its diagnosis is lacking

Summary

General personality disorder (PD) criteria (G1–G6) *must* be fulfilled before a specific personality disorder is diagnosed
BAD CROACk

F60.0 Paranoid PD
SUSPECTS

F60.1 Schizoid PD
PECULIARS

F60.2 Dissocial PD
CRIMES

F60.30 Impulsive type
SCOLD

F60.31 Borderline type
PLEAS

F60.4 Histrionic PD
PRAISE

F60.5 Anankastic PD
SLOW FIRM

F60.6 Anxious (avoidant) PD
CRIKEY

F60.7 Dependent PD
DEPEND

F63.0 Pathological gambling
2 PoUND (think cash/£)

F63.1 Pathological fire-setting (pyromania)
2 PUFF (think puff of smoke)

F63.2 Pathological stealing (kleptomania)
2 US (thieves steal from us)

F63.3 Trichotillomania
NULL (left with little/null hair)

F64.0 Transsexualism
Note the 'sex' part, i.e. gender – where an individual wishes to live as a member of the opposite sex

F64.1 Dual-role transvestism
= *vest*/clothing

F64.2 Gender identity disorder of childhood
GID

F65 Disorders of sexual preference
ODD

Chapter 8

Mental retardation/learning disability (F70–F79)

This equates to a condition of arrested or incomplete development of the mind, characterised by an impairment of skills manifested during the developmental period, which contributes to the overall level of intelligence, i.e. cognitive, language, motor and social abilities. The diagnosis is made by clinical and psychometric assessment and current levels of functioning.

Two main components of mental retardation (MR)/learning disability:
1. Level of *cognitive* abilities
2. Level of *social* competence (the Vineland Social Maturity Scale can be used to assess this)
N.B. It is important to consider cultural and social issues in clinical assessments

The fourth character provides subdivisions to identify the extent of impairment of behaviour:
.0 no/minimal impairment of behaviour
.1 significant impairment of behaviour requiring attention/treatment
.8 other impairments of behaviour
.9 without mention of impairment of behaviour

Coding

Approximate IQ score range (for both ICD-10 and DSM-IV):
Mild MR 50–69
Moderate MR 35–49
Severe MR 20–34
Profound MR <20
Note: **O MUMPS** (*see p.6*)

Usually tested via the Wechsler Adult Intelligence Scale in adults

Mild F70 – in adults the mental age is 9–12 years, some learning difficulties identified at school. Adults are usually able to work and maintain social relationships

Moderate F71 – in adults, the mental age is 6–9 years. There are marked developmental delays in childhood. Most are able to have some independence in self-care and acquire adequate communication and academic skills

Severe F72 – in adults, the mental age is 3–6 years. They are likely to require full-time support

Profound F73 – in adults, the mental age is less than three years old. There is severe limitation in self-care, continence, communication and mobility

Other mental retardation, F78

Unspecified mental retardation, F79

Chapter 9

Disorders of psychological development (F80–F89)

Onset is in infancy or childhood and is associated with central nervous system maturation. These disorders are not associated with episodic deterioration. The functions affected include language, visuo-spatial skills and co-ordination

F80 Specific developmental disorders of speech and language

Language acquisition is delayed
Often associated with reading and spelling problems, interpersonal relationships and emotional and behavioural disorders
'Specific' suggests only that particular disorder is present

F80.0 Specific speech articulation disorder
The child's *use of speech sounds* is <u>below</u> the appropriate level for their mental age
Language skills are within normal limits

F80.1 Expressive language disorder
The child's *use of expressive spoken language* is <u>below</u> the appropriate level for their mental age
Comprehension of language is within normal limits

F80.2 Receptive language disorder
The child's *understanding of language* is <u>below</u> the appropriate level for their mental age
Expressive language is also affected and abnormalities in word–sound production are frequent problems
Mixed receptive/expressive disorder

F80.3 Acquired aphasia with epilepsy (Landau–Kleffner syndrome)

A child (usually aged 3–7 years), who has made normal progress in language skills, loses both receptive and expressive language skills
Normal intelligence is retained and the onset is associated with a characteristic EEG and epileptic seizures
Two-thirds of patients are left with a severe receptive language deficit

Two-thirds left with RLD (receptive language deficit)
Intelligence normal
Loss of skills (receptive and expressive language skills)
EEG/epileptic seizures

TILE

F80.8 Other developmental disorders of speech and language

Includes *lisping*

F80.9 Developmental disorder of speech and language, unspecified

Language disorder NOS

F81 Specific developmental disorder of scholastic skills

Normal patterns of skill acquisition are affected from early development

F81.0 Specific reading disorder
For example, developmental dyslexia
Reading skills acquisition disorder
Not accounted for by mental age, visual acuity, neurological disorder and poor schooling
Associated emotional and behavioural problems are common
Preceded by disorders of language or speech development

Reading skills acquisition that interferes with academic achievements or activities of daily living
Exclusions noted (as above), for example, visual, educational, IQ or neurological problems
Associated (preceding) emotional and behavioural problems are common
Disorders of language/speech development common

READ

F81.1 Specific spelling disorder
Specific spelling disorder – oral and written
Present from early stages of development
Exclusions – specific reading disorder, visual acuity problems, IQ <70
Little evidence of inadequacies in educational experiences
Limits overall academic achievement and activities of daily living

SPELL

F81.2 Specific disorder of arithmetical skills
Involves a specific impairment in arithmetical skills not related purely to a low IQ or poor schooling

F81.3 Mixed disorder of scholastic skills
This is a residual category where both arithmetical and reading or spelling are affected
Learning disability and poor schooling are exclusions

F81.8 Other developmental disorders of scholastic skills
Developmental expressive writing disorder

F81.9 Developmental disorder of scholastic skills, unspecified
NOS disorders

F82 Specific developmental disorder of motor function

Serious impairment in the development of motor co-ordination that is not purely related to general learning disability or any neurological disorder. There is evidence of neurodevelopmental immaturities and interference with daily activities or academic achievement

F83 Mixed specific developmental disorders

A residual category for mixtures of specific developmental disorders of speech and language/scholastic skills/motor function

F84 Pervasive developmental disorders

Abnormalities in:

Social interactions
Stereotyped repertoire of interests and activities
Speech/communication
Across all **S**ituations

4 × S

F84.0 Childhood autism
Atypical/impaired development noted before the **A**ge of three years
Reciprocal **S**ocial interactions
Communication/**S**peech
Restricted, **S**tereotyped behaviour, interests or activities
Frequent **E**motional/**B**ehavioural difficulties: phobias, sleeping, eating, temper and aggression difficulties

Behavioural difficulties
Age <3 years when difficulties in development are noted
Social interactions/speech/stereotyped behaviours
Emotional difficulties

BAS₃E

F84.1 Atypical autism

Abnormal development is notable at/after **T**hree years old
Social interactions/**S**peech/**S**tereotyped behaviours
Does not meet the criteria for **A**utism

Social interactions/speech/stereotyped behaviours
Autism criteria unmet
Three years (abnormal development at/after 3 years)

S₃AT

F84.10 Atypicality in age of onset

F84.11 Atypicality in symptomatology

F84.12 Atypicality in both age of onset and symptomatology

F84.2 Rett's syndrome

Girls – occurs in the female gender
Onset 7–24 months
Loss of speech (expressive and receptive language disorder) and locomotion (stereotyped hand movements)
Development (early) normal
Deceleration in head growth

GOLD₂

F84.3 Other childhood disintegrative disorder

A type of pervasive developmental disorder

Stereotyped repetitive motor mannerisms
Knowledge and skills are intact up to the age of at least two years, i.e. normal development up to two years
Autism-like abnormalities in social **I**nteraction + communication
Loss of skills over several months
Loss of interest in the environment

SKILL

F84.4 Overactive disorder associated with mental retardation and stereotyped movements
Severe motor **H**yperactivity (e.g. including restlessness, difficulties in remaining seated, rapid changes in activity, repeated motor mannerisms, risky behaviour (self-harm))
Absent autistic features, i.e. social impairment of the autistic type
Ill-defined disorder
LQ is less than 50 (**L**earning disability)

HAIL

F84.5 Asperger's syndrome
Similar to autism (with regard to social interaction, restricted, stereotyped repertoire of interests) but *no* global delay or retardation, delay in language or cognitive development
Often marked **C**lumsiness
Abnormalities **P**ersist into adulthood
Occasional psychotic episodes in early adult life
Exclude other varieties of pervasive developmental disorder such as simple schizophrenia or personality disorders

SCOPE

F84.8 Other pervasive developmental disorders

F84.9 Pervasive developmental disorder unspecified
A category used when an individual fits a diagnosis of pervasive developmental disorder but there is either contradictory information or inadequate information to justify the diagnosis of F84

F88 Other disorders of psychological development

For example, developmental agnosia

F89 Unspecified disorder of psychological development

For example, developmental disorder, NOS

Summary

F80.3 Acquired aphasia with epilepsy (Landau–Kleffner syndrome)
TILE

F81.0 Specific reading disorder
READ

F81.1 Specific spelling disorder
SPELL

F84 Pervasive developmental disorders
4 x S

F84.0 Childhood autism
BAS$_3$E

F84.1 Atypical autism
S$_3$AT

F84.2 Rett's syndrome
GOLD$_2$

F84.3 Other childhood disintegrative disorder
SKILL

F84.4 Overactive disorder associated with mental retardation and stereotyped movements
HAIL

F84.5 Asperger's syndrome
SCOPE

Chapter 10

Behavioural and emotional disorders with onset usually occurring in childhood and adolescence (F90–F99)

F90 Hyperkinetic disorders

G1 Inattention – symptoms have persisted for six months to a problematic level and not consistent with the child's development

G2 Hyperactivity – maladaptive + inconsistent with development for six months

G3 Impulsivity – maladaptive + inconsistent with development for six months

G4 Onset no later than seven years old

G5 Pervasive – occurs across a range of situations

G6 G1–G3 cause significant distress

G7 Does not meet criteria for pervasive developmental disorders, manic episode, depressive episode or anxiety disorders

Seven years – onset no later than this age + **S**ocial distress
Hyperactivity
Impulsivity + **I**nattention
Pervasive

SHIP

F90.0 Disturbance of activity and attention
Attention deficit:
– Disorder with hyperactivity
– Hyperactivity disorder
– Syndrome with hyperactivity

F90.1 Hyperkinetic conduct disorder
Both Hyperkinetic disorder and Conduct disorder criteria must be met for this category

F90.8 Other hyperkinetic disorders

F90.9 Hyperkinetic disorder NOS
A residual category when F90.0 and F90.1 are extremely similar, but the overall criteria for F90.– are fulfilled

F91 Conduct disorder (CD)

A repetitive, persistent pattern of dissocial, defiant and aggressive conduct
An enduring pattern of behaviour lasting six months or more
Exclude other psychiatric disorders – affective disorder, pervasive developmental disorder, schizophrenia or hyperkinetic disorder

Conduct problems, i.e. behaviour
Rule violation
Onset is specified
Six months' duration
Symptoms not attributable to another mental disorder

CROSS

Examples include:

Fighting
Arson, Acquisitive offences
Truanting
Animal cruelty, arguments
Lying

FATAL

Specify age of onset

Childhood onset: at least one conduct problem before 10 years old
Adolescent onset: no conduct problems before 10 years old

Context

Socialised – presence of lasting peer friendships
Unsocialised – absence of lasting peer friendships
Familial – confined to the family context

Dimensions of disturbance

Hyperactivity (e.g. restless behaviour or inattention)
Emotional disturbance (anxiety, depression, hypochondriasis, obsessionality)
Severity: mild/moderate or severe

F91.0 Conduct disorder confined to the family context
Meets the general criteria for CD
3/more of the (FATAL) symptoms listed in the above criteria
Duration six months
Limited to the family context

F91.1 Unsocialised CD
Meets the general criteria for CD
3/more of the (FATAL) symptoms listed in the above criteria
Duration at least six months
Definite poor relationships with <u>the individual's peer group</u> – isolation/
rejection/unpopularity/lack of close reciprocal relationships

F91.2 Socialised CD
Meets the general criteria for CD
3/more of the (FATAL) symptoms listed in the above criteria
Duration at least six months
Includes settings other than house or family environment
Peer relationships are within normal limits

F91.3 Oppositional defiant disorder
Meets the general criteria for CD
Usually seen in *younger* children than CD
4/more of the (FATAL) symptoms listed in the above criteria
Maladaptive + unrelated to the developmental level
Duration at least six months

F91.8 Other CD

F91.9 Conduct disorder, unspecified
Residual category – when unfulfilled by other subtypes

F92 Mixed disorders of conduct and emotions

F92.0 Depressive conduct disorder

General criteria for CD (F91) met + criteria for one affective disorder met (F30–F39)

F92.8 Other mixed disorders of conduct and emotions

General criteria for CD (F91) met + criteria for neurotic, stress-related and somatoform disorder (F40–F48) or childhood emotional disorder (F93) are met

F92.9 Mixed disorder of conduct and emotions, unspecified

F93 Emotional disorders with onset specific to childhood

Usually developmental milestones are normal and emotional responses are exaggerations of normal states

F93.0 Separation anxiety disorder of childhood

Sleep disturbance as a result of separation at night
Exclude generalised anxiety disorder of childhood
Physical symptoms in response to separation
Alone – fear of being alone
Repeated school refusal
Anxiety about separation or harm befalling main attachment figures
Time – onset before the age of six years
Exclude emotion, conduct, personality disorders or pervasive developmental disorder (PDD)
Distressed and duration at least four weeks

SEPARATED

F93.1 Phobic anxiety disorder of childhood

Phobia: (a persistent fear) which causes a significant social impairment
Occurs for at least four weeks
Beyond normal worries
Impairment (socially)
Criteria for other disorders (such as generalised anxiety disorder) are unmet

PhOBIC

F93.2 Social anxiety disorder of childhood (SADOC)

Socially awkward and avoidant
Anxiety about self-appropriateness
Duration of at least four weeks
Onset before six years
Criteria for generalised anxiety disorder of childhood unmet

SADOC

F93.3 Sibling rivalry

Negative feelings toward sibling
Emotional disturbance, e.g. tantrums, sleep problems
Six months of the birth of the sibling
Time – at least four weeks

NEST

F93.8 Other childhood emotional disorders
Includes Identity disorder and Over-anxious disorder

F93.80 Generalised anxiety disorder (GAD) of childhood

General symptoms – restlessness, irritability, tiredness, muscle tension, etc. across a variety of different situations
Anxiety and worries over at least two situations, activities, contexts or circumstances
Difficult to control the worry and distress over six months

GAD

F93.9 Childhood emotional disorder, unspecified

F94 Disorders of social functioning with onset specific to childhood and adolescence

F94.0 Elective mutism

Marked selectivity in speaking (usually in specific social interactions)
Understands language (normal language expression and comprehension)
Time – duration lasts longer than four weeks
Exclude PDD, or a specific speech or language disorder

MUTE

F94.1 Reactive attachment disorder of childhood

Remove this diagnosis: if PDD present
Emotional disturbance – lack of emotional responsiveness, withdrawal, aggression to the child's own/others' distress, and/or hypervigilance
Ambivalent social responses
Capacity for social interactions is evidenced
Time – onset before the age of five years

REACT

F94.2 Disinhibited attachment disorder of childhood

Diffuse attachments within the first five years of life
Inappropriate social interactions with strangers
Selective social interactions
Clingy in infancy
Overly attention seeking and indiscriminately friendly, in early to middle childhood

DISCO

F94.8 Other childhood disorders of social functioning

F94.9 Childhood disorder of social functioning, unspecified

F95 Tic disorders

F95.0 Transient tic disorder

Tics occur before the age of 18 years

Involves four weeks of symptoms

Continues for *a year or less*

Side-effects of medications, history of Tourette's or medical conditions are exclusions

TICS

F95.1 Chronic tic disorder

Tics occur before the age of 18 years

Includes a maximum of two months remission over a year

Continues for *a year or more*

Side-effects of medications, history of Tourette's or medical conditions are exclusions

F95.8 Other tic disorders

F95.9 Tic disorder, unspecified

F98 Other behavioural and emotional disorders with onset occurring in childhood and adolescence

F98.0 Non-organic enuresis
Seven years old – used as a diagnostic cut-off, based on symptoms*
Time – three months' duration at least
Age (mental age and chronological age – at least four years old)
Involuntary or intentional socially inappropriate voiding
Not a consequence of an underlying medical condition
Separate this from any other mental disorder (exclusions)

STAINS
Voiding occurs at least twice a month in children aged under seven years and at least once a month in children aged seven and above.

F98.1 Non-organic encopresis
Faeces 'flow'– repeated intentional/involuntary passage of this
Age (mental age and chronological age – at least four years old)
Encopretic event occurs every month
Continues for at least six months
Exclude an organic cause
Socially inappropriate places used for defaecating

FAECES

F98.2 Feeding disorder of infancy and childhood
Fails to gain/loses weight over at least one month
Exclude any other organic or mental disorder
Eating disorder – fails to eat adequately or ruminates or regurgitates food
Disorder occurs before…
Six years old

FEEDS

F98.3 Pica of infancy and childhood
Pica sounds like '*picks at*'

Persistent eating of non-nutritive substances, at least twice a week
In one month (at least)
Criteria for other conditions unmet and Culture inappropriate
Age (mental age and chronological age – at least two years old)

PICA

F98.4 Stereotyped movement disorder (SMD)
Stereotyped movements – lead to significant distress
Mental retardation/learning disability common
Duration at least one month

SMD

F98.5 Stuttering
Speech includes frequent repetition/prolongation/syllables/words affecting speech rhythm
Three syllables (in stuttering) = three-month duration (at least)

F98.6 Cluttering
Rapid speech – no repetition or hesitation
Three syllables in Cluttering = three-month duration (at least)

F98.8 Other specified behavioural and emotional disorders with onset usually occurring in childhood and adolescence

F98.9 Unspecified behavioural and emotional disorders with onset usually occurring in childhood and adolescence

F99 Mental disorder, not otherwise specified
Non-recommended 'residual' category

Summary

F90 Hyperkinetic disorders
SHIP

F91 Conduct disorder
FATAL CROSS

F93 Separation anxiety disorder of childhood
SEPARATED

F93.1 Phobic anxiety disorder of childhood
PhOBIC

F93.2 Social anxiety disorder of childhood (SADOC)
SADOC

F93.3 Sibling rivalry
NEST

F93.80 Generalised anxiety disorder of childhood
GAD

F94.0 Elective mutism
MUTE

F94.1 Reactive attachment disorder of childhood
REACT

F94.2 Disinhibited attachment disorder of childhood
DISCO

F95.0 Transient tic disorder
TICS

F98.0 Non-organic eneuresis
STAINS

F98.1 Non-organic encopresis
FAECES

F98.2 Feeding disorder of infancy and childhood
FEEDS

F98.3 Pica of infancy and childhood
PICA

F98.4 Stereotyped movement disorder
SMD

Chapter 11
Culture-specific disorders

These are listed *separately* from the body of the main ICD-10 codes, but are present within ICD-10

Amok

Amnesia/fatigue follows episode
Menacing behaviour/**M**alayan origin
Out of the blue
Kamikaze – often leads to suicide

AMOK

Possible ICD-10 coding:
F68.8   Other specific disorders of adult personality and behaviour

Dhat

Decrease in semen (concern)
Heralded by a change in routine/diet/genitourinary disorders
Anxiety
Tension (muscular)

DHAT

Possible ICD-10 coding:
F45.34 Somatoform autonomic dysfunction of the genitourinary system
F48.8   Other specified neurotic disorders

Koro

Known precursors including excess coitus/cold exposure/illness or interpersonal stress
Ominous outcome – fear of death
Retraction of genitals
Onset rapid

KORO

Possible ICD-10 code:
F45.34 Somatoform autonomic dysfunction of the genitourinary system
F48.8   Other specified neurotic disorders

Latah

Low self-esteem in sufferers
Amusing experience for onlookers
Tends to occur in Malaysian women primarily
Adverse experience for sufferers
Highly exaggerated responses to arousal stimulus – echolalia/echopraxia/trance-like state

LATAH

Possible ICD-10 code:
F44.88 Other specified dissociative (conversion) disorders
F48.8   Other specified neurotic disorders

Nerfiza, nerves, nevra, nervios

Nausea
Episodic, chronic anxiety/sorrow
Reactivity reduced
Vigilance – poor sleep
Excitement/agitation
Somatic complaints

NERVES

Possible ICD-10 code:
F32.11 Moderate depressive episode with somatic syndrome
F45.1　Undifferentiated somatoform disorder
F48.0　Neurasthenia

Pa-leng, frigophobia

Think: *Fridge*: Frigo, i.e. fear of cold
Feelings of anxiety that coldness can lead to death

Possible ICD-10 code:
F40.2　Specific phobias

Pibloktoq, Arctic hysteria

Prodromal fatigue
Inuit populations (Arctic)
Behaviours follow including seizure type
Loss of consciousness
Only a few minutes in duration then a full recovery follows

PIBLO

Possible ICD-10 code:
F44.7　Mixed dissociative (conversion) disorders
F44.88 Other specified dissociative (conversion) disorders

Susto, espanto

Soul loss fear
Upset if others are distressed
Supernatural fright induced
Temperature can be raised (fever)
Overactive conscious state – agitation, anorexia, insomnia, mental confusion, apathy, depression

SUSTO

Possible ICD-10 code
F45.1   Undifferentiated somatoform disorder
F48.8   Other specified neurotic disorder

Taijin kyofusho, shinkeishitsu, anthropophobia

Japanese in origin
Fear of social contact
Variety of somatic complaints
Extreme self-consciousness, and a fear of contracting disease
Think ANTH from anthropophobia (fear of people)

Anxiety state with somatic complaints
Negative self-image
Timid – fear of social contact
Hypochondriachal thoughts

ANTH

Possible ICD-10 code:
F40.1   Social phobia
F40.8   Other phobic anxiety disorders

Ufufuyane, saka

Spirit possession
Anxiety state
Known to be provoked by the sight of men or foreigners
Attacks last days to weeks

SAKA
*Note: SA*ka – South Africa originating

Possible ICD-10 code:
F44.3   Trance and possession disorders
F44.7   Mixed dissociative (conversion) disorders

Uqamairineq

Sudden paralysis associated with borderline sleep states
Often accompanied by anxiety, agitation and hallucinations
Usually chronic, can be acute
Lasts minutes and felt to be caused by the 'soul wandering'
Seen in Inuits living within the Arctic Circle

SOULS

Possible ICD-10 code:
F44.88 Other specified dissociative (conversion) disorders
F47.4   Narcolepsy and cataplexy
Includes: sleep paralysis

Windigo

Wild/cannibalistic obsessive behaviour
Includes other symptoms: depression, homicidal or suicidal thoughts,
and a delusional compulsive wish to eat human flesh
NE USA native population
Domain of history – mostly historic accounts

WIND

Possible ICD-10 code:
F68.8   Other specified disorders of personality and behaviour

Summary

Amok
AMOK

Dhat
DHAT

Koro
KORO

Latah
LATAH

Nerfiza, nerves, nevra, nervios
NERVES

Pa-leng, frigophobia
Think: *Fridge*: Frigo, i.e. fear of cold

Pibloktoq, Arctic hysteria
PIBLO

Susto, espanto
SUSTO

Taijin kyofusho, shinkeishitsu, anthropophobia
ANTH

Ufufuyane, saka
SAKA

Uqamairineq
SOULS

Windigo
WIND

Chapter 12
Miscellaneous disorders

This includes those disorders whose significance, either scientific or clinical, remains uncertain within the ICD-10

Seasonal affective disorder

Seasonal affective episodes outnumber any non-seasonal episodes
Always occur within a particular 90-day period (both episodes and remissions)
Duration – three episodes occurring at the same time of year for three or more consecutive years

SAD

N.B. *Three* letters in SAD... similar to the duration (in years) for SAD
Can be applied to F30–F33 affective disorders

Bipolar II disorder

Bipolar II is numerically $\underline{H}$igher than bipolar I – $\underline{H}$*ypomania* rather than mania

A. 1/ more episodes of depression (F32.-)
B. 1/ more episodes of hypomania (F30.0)
C. No episodes of mania (F30.1-F30.2)
(Applies to bipolar affective disorder: F31.0. F31.3–F31.5, F31.7)

Rapid cycling bipolar disorder

F31.0–F31.7
The criteria for bipolar affective disorder (F31.0–F31.7) must be fulfilled
At least four episodes of bipolar affective disorder must occur within a 12-month period.
Rapid cycling bipolar disorder = four words: four months

Narcissistic personality disorder

The general criteria for personality disorder must be fulfilled (F60)
Five of the following:

Grandiose sense of self-importance
Recognition of others' emotion is not present
Exploitation of interpersonal relationships
Arrogance in behaviours and attitudes
Treatment from others has to be favourable
Envy of others or feeling that others are envious
Excessive admiration required
Special + unique
Thoughts of self-importance

GREATE$_2$ST

Passive-aggressive (negativistic) personality disorder

The general criteria for personality disorder must be fulfilled (F60)
At least five of the following:

Procrastination in completing tasks
Avoidance of obligations through forgetfulness
Sulkiness when asked to do something not wanted
Slow or poor work deliberately
Impedes the efforts of others by not doing their work
Vitriolic towards those in authority
Expostulation/objection of others' unreasonable demands

PASSIVE

Summary

Seasonal affective disorder
SAD

Bipolar II disorder
Bipolar II is _H_igher than bipolar I – _Hypomania_ rather than mania

Rapid cycling bipolar disorder
Rapid cycling bipolar disorder = four words: four months

Narcissistic personality disorder
GREATEST

Passive-aggressive personality disorder
PASSIVE

Index